FOOD TRACKER

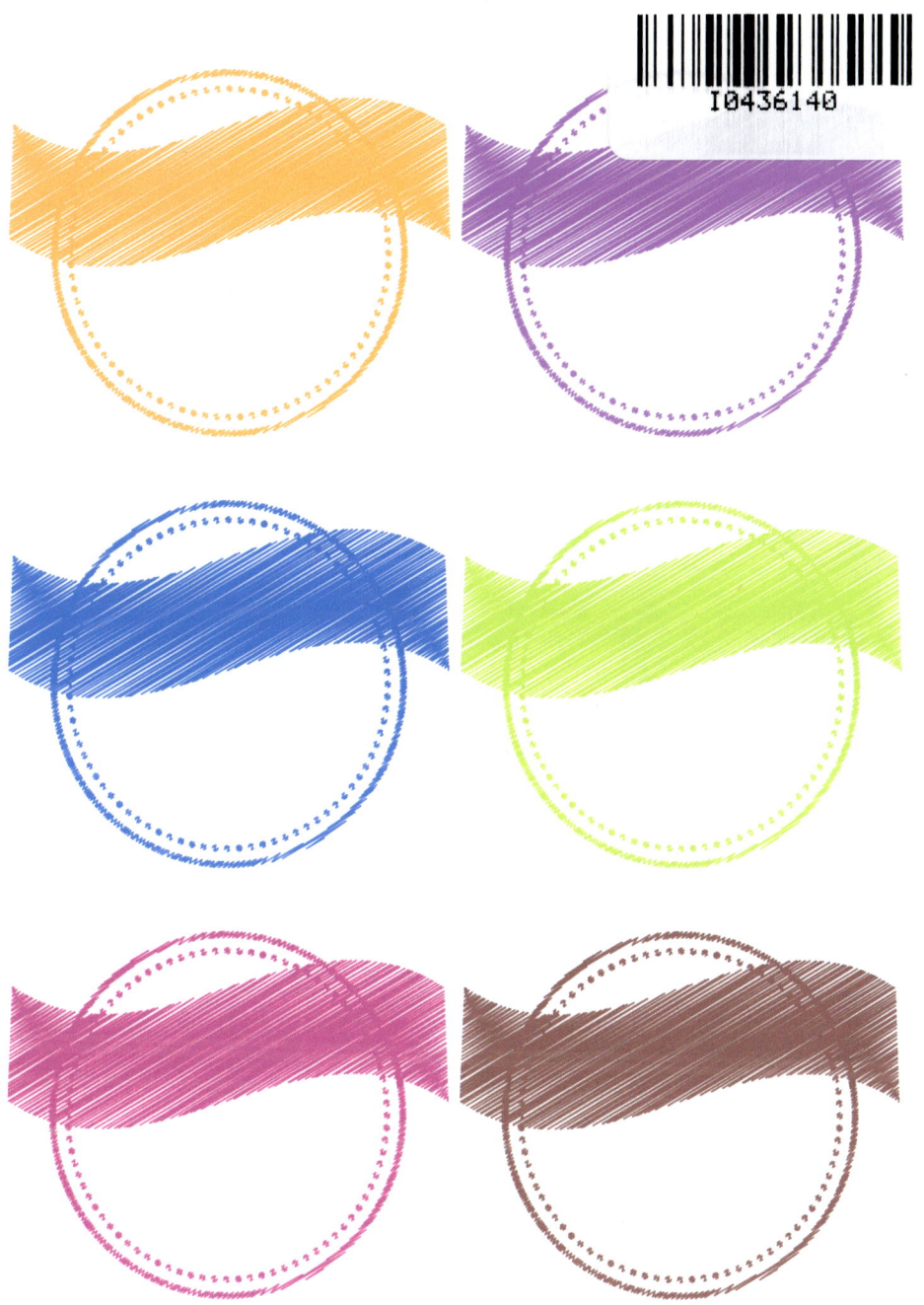

FOOD TRACKER

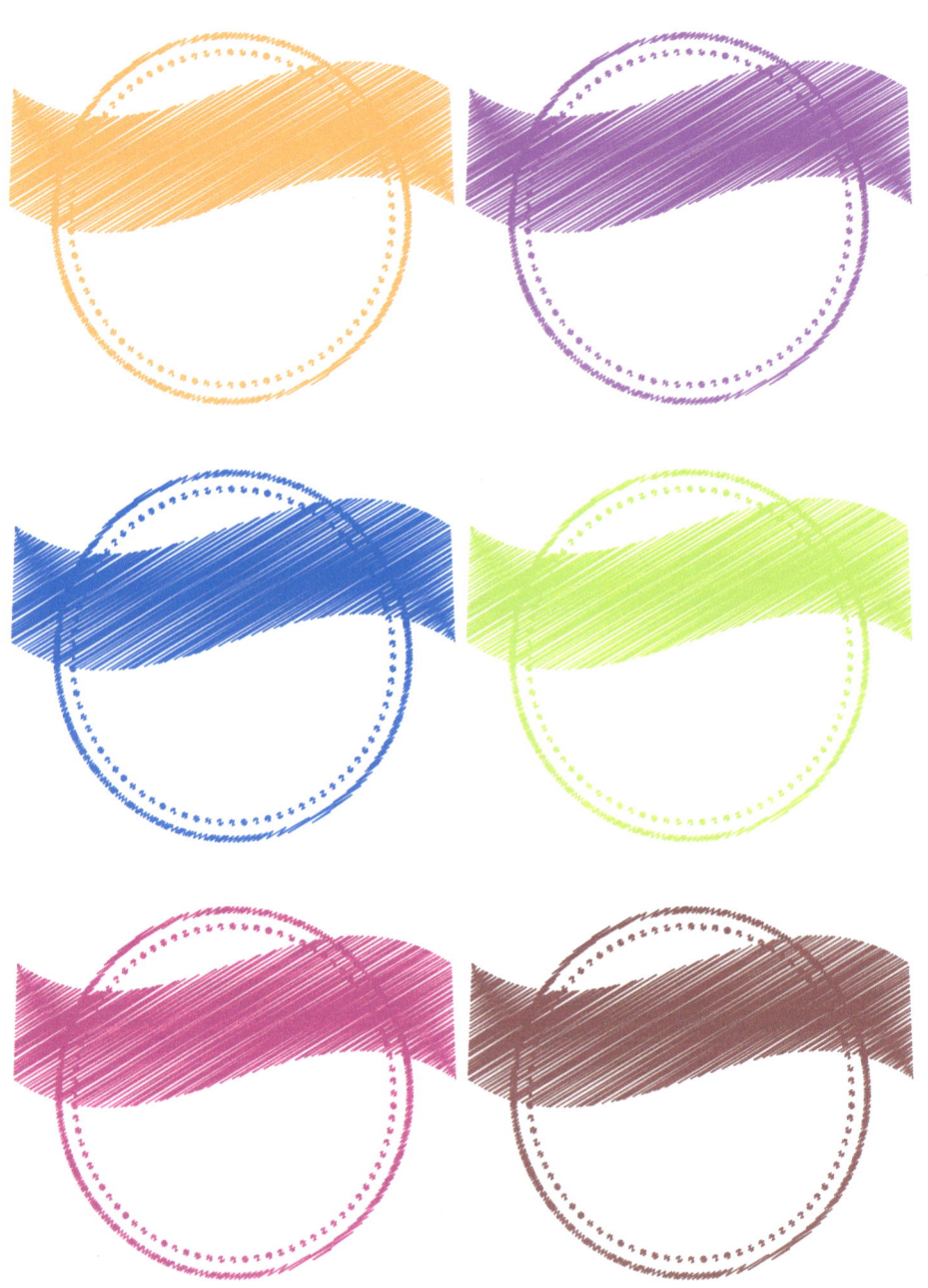

FOOD TRACKER

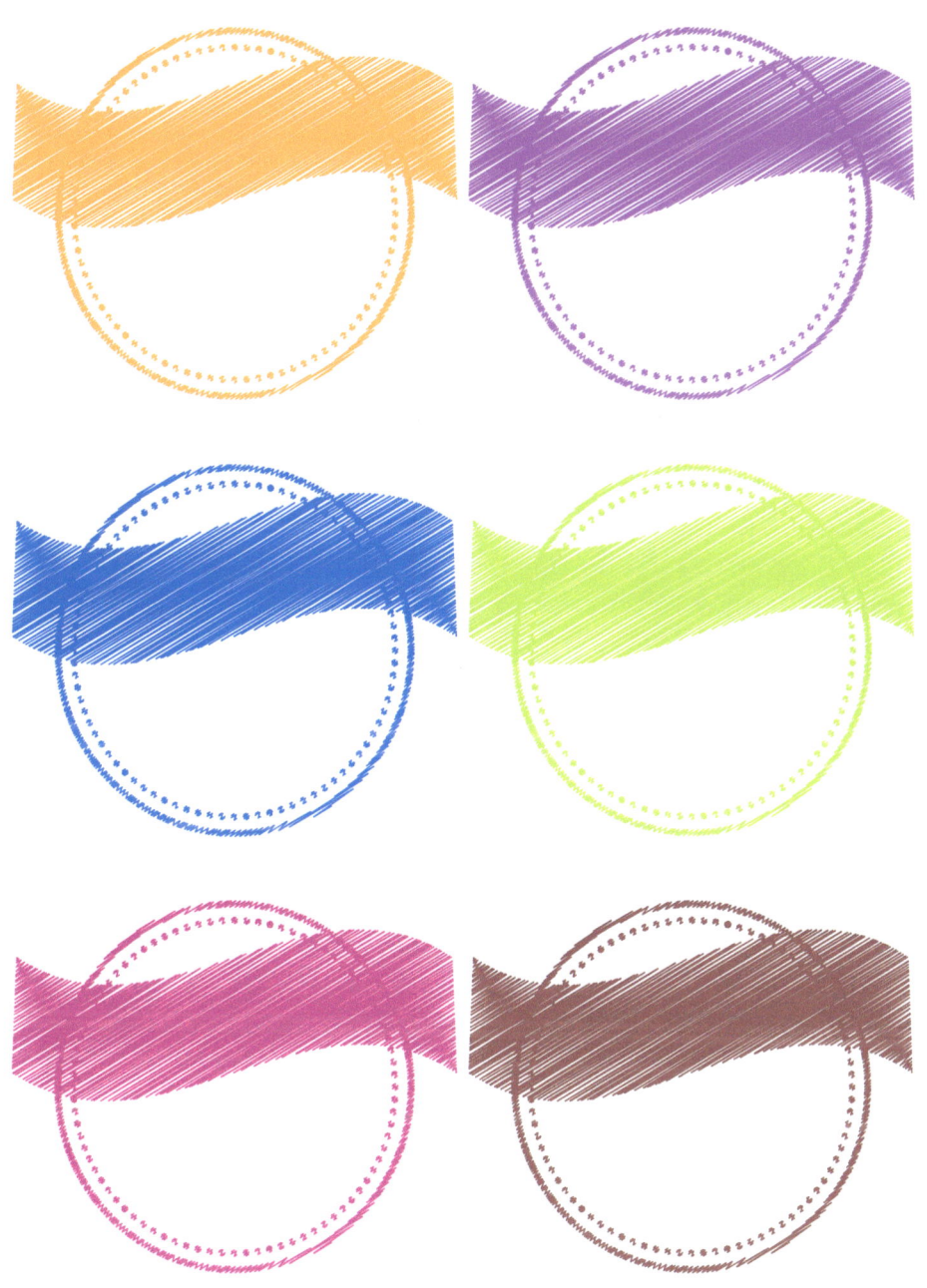

FOOD TRACKER

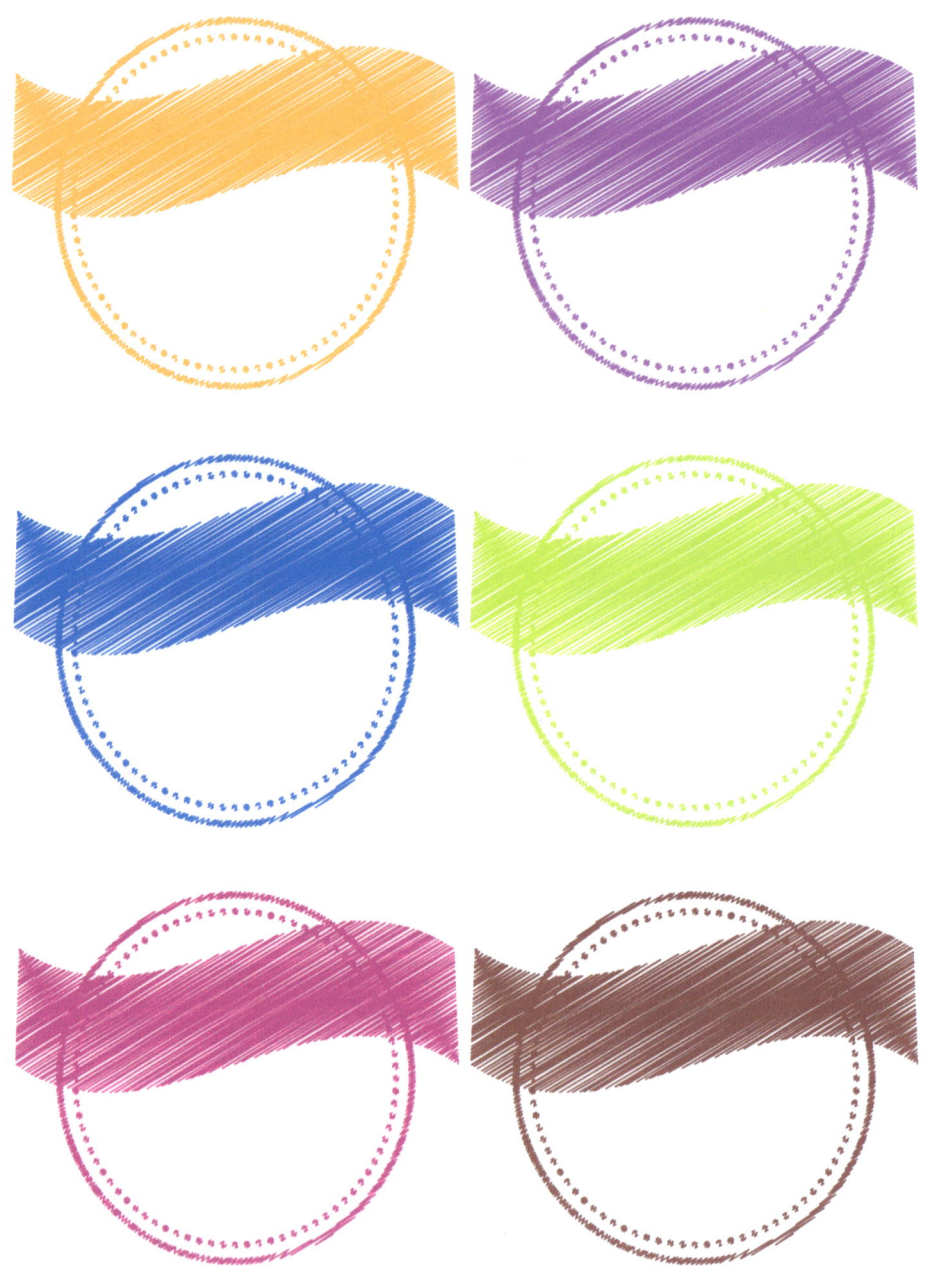

FOOD TRACKER

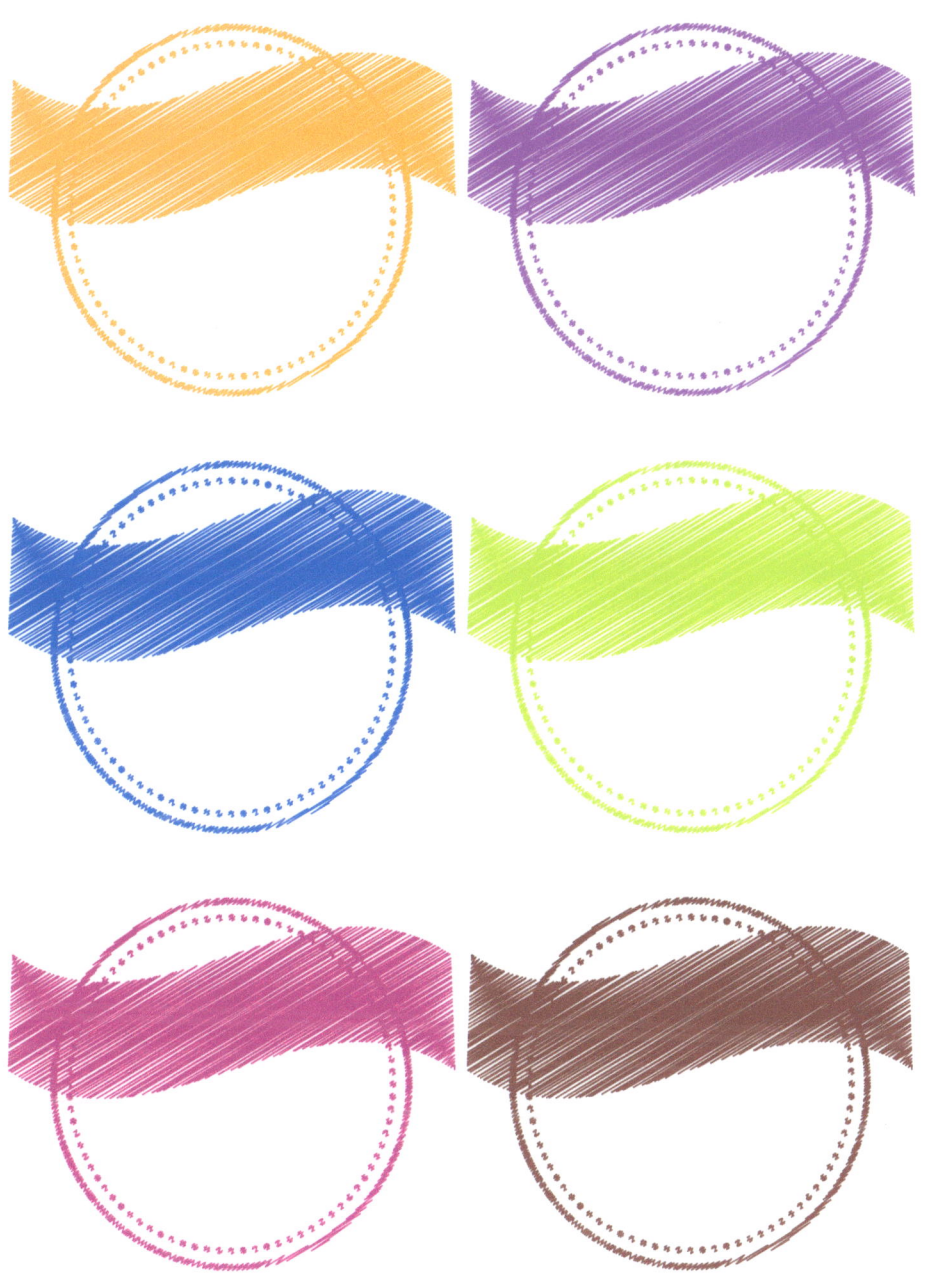

FOOD TRACKER

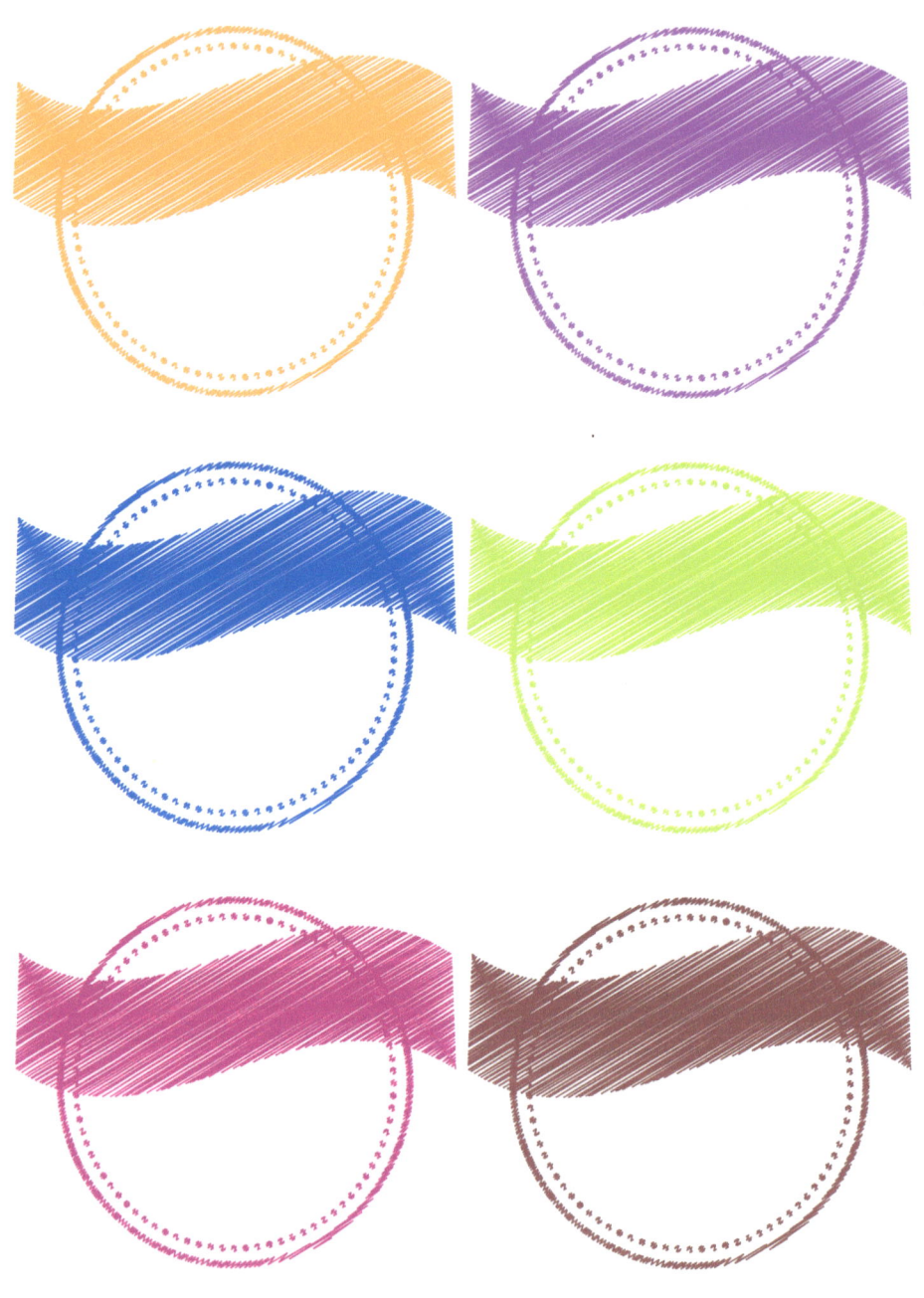

FOOD TRACKER

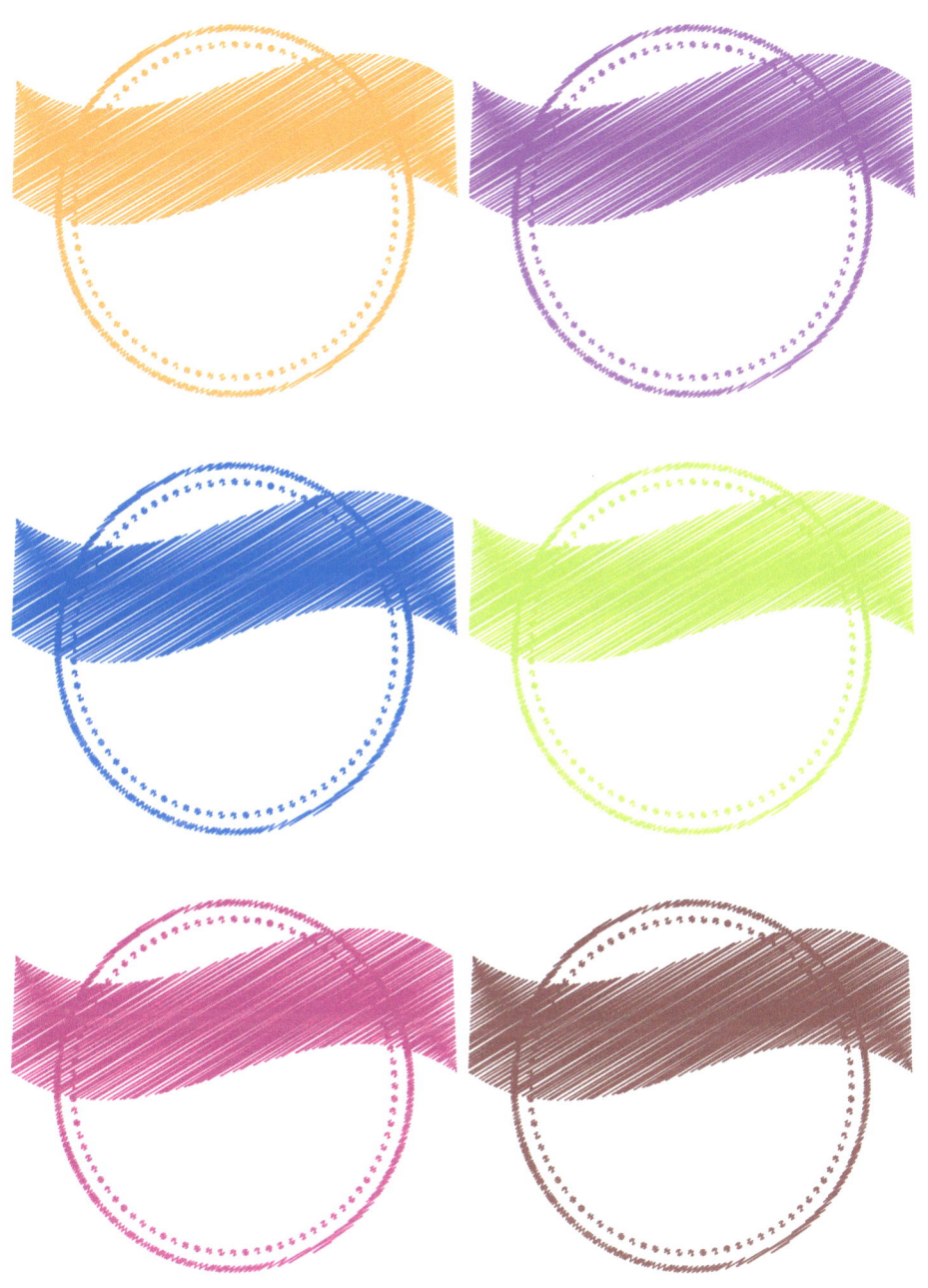

FOOD TRACKER

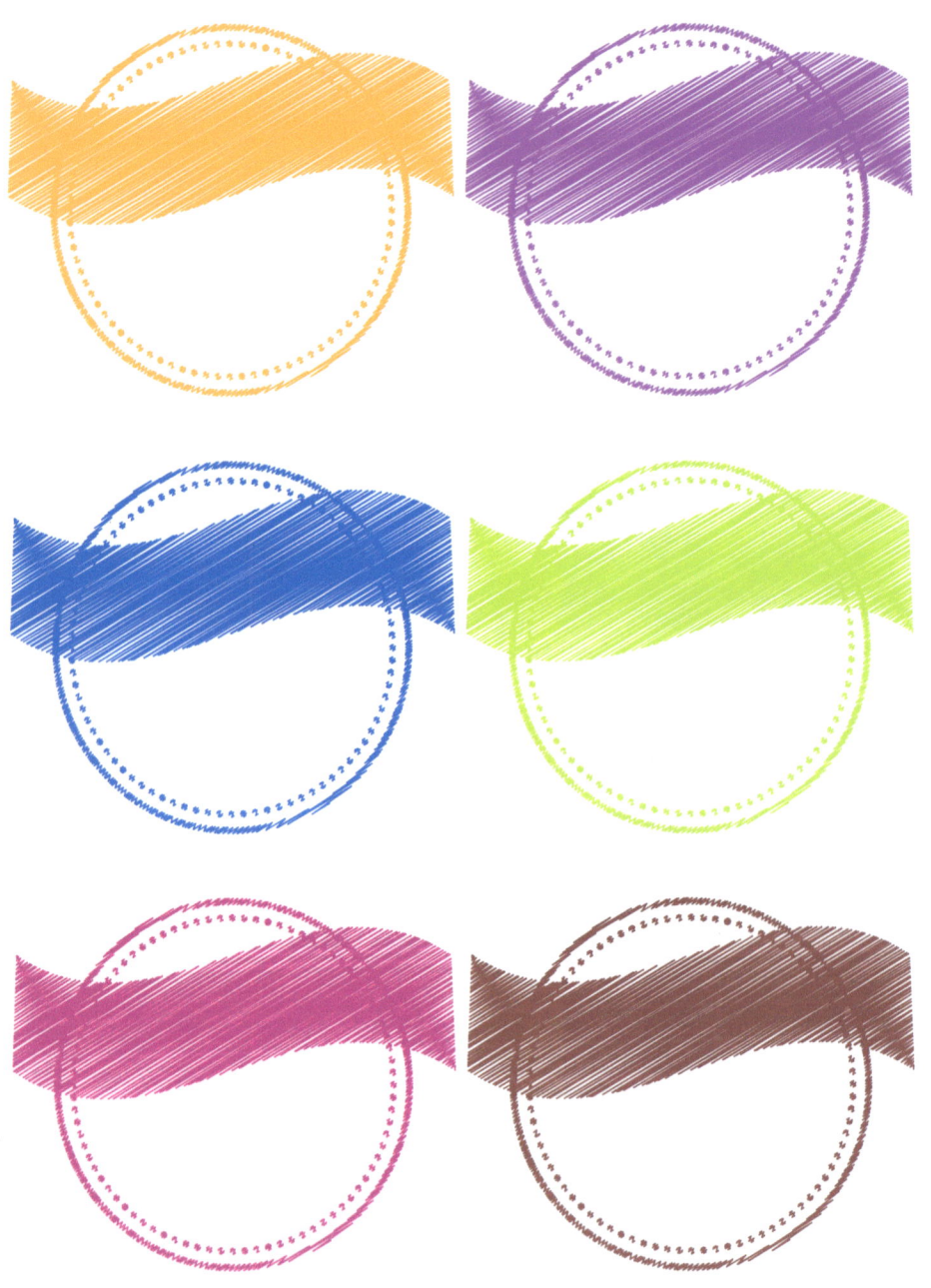

FOOD TRACKER

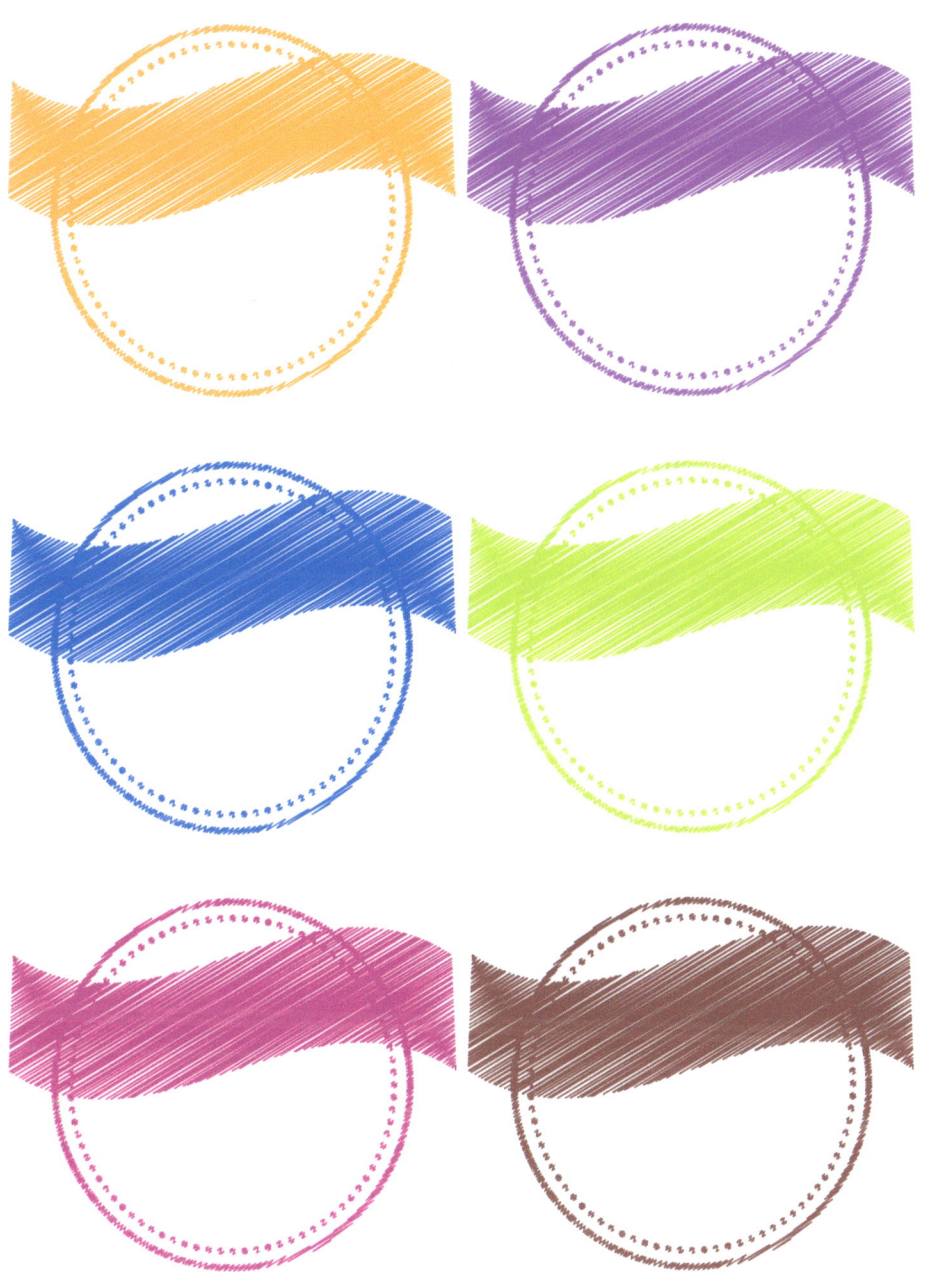

FOOD TRACKER

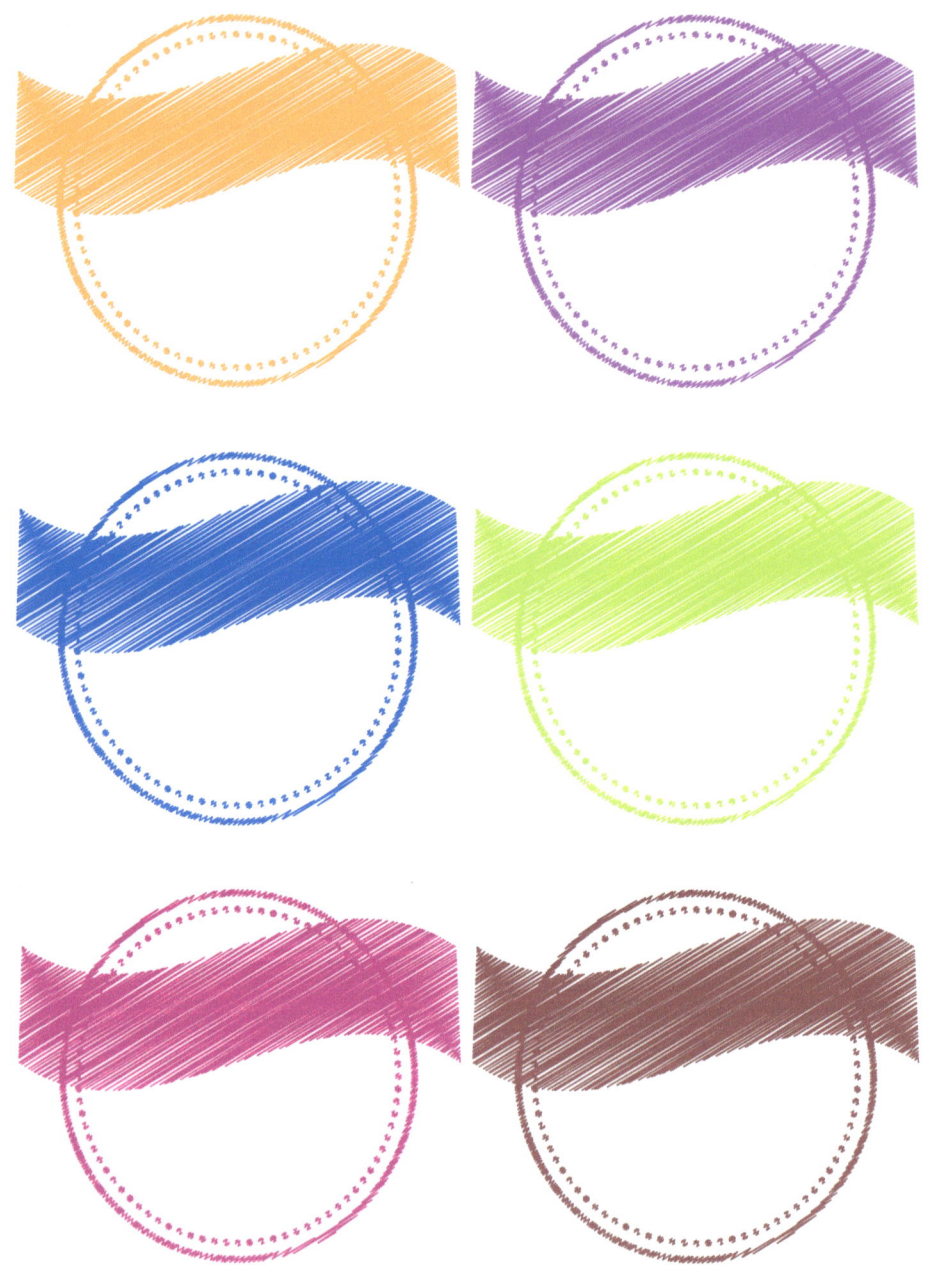

FOOD TRACKER

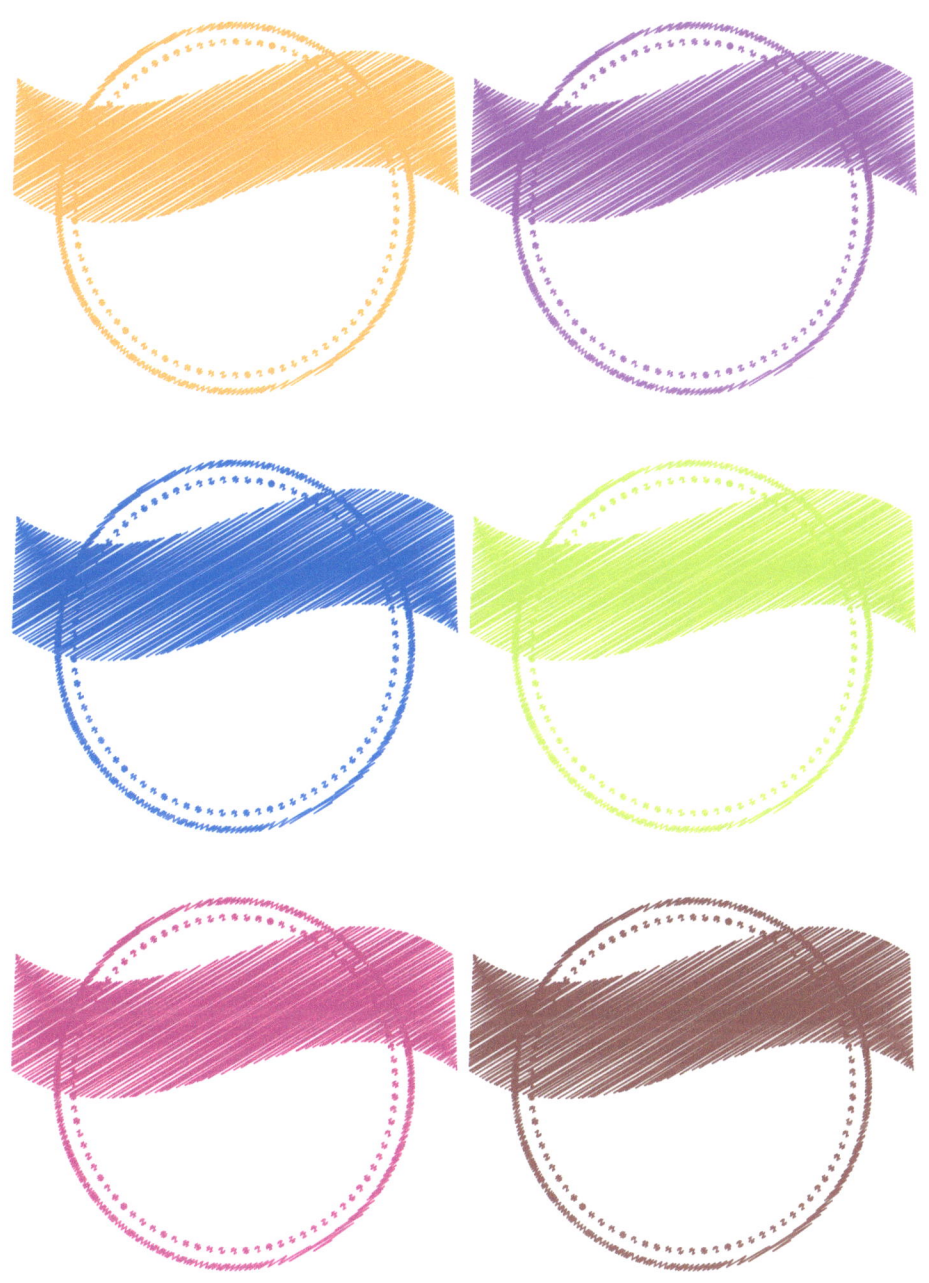

FOOD TRACKER

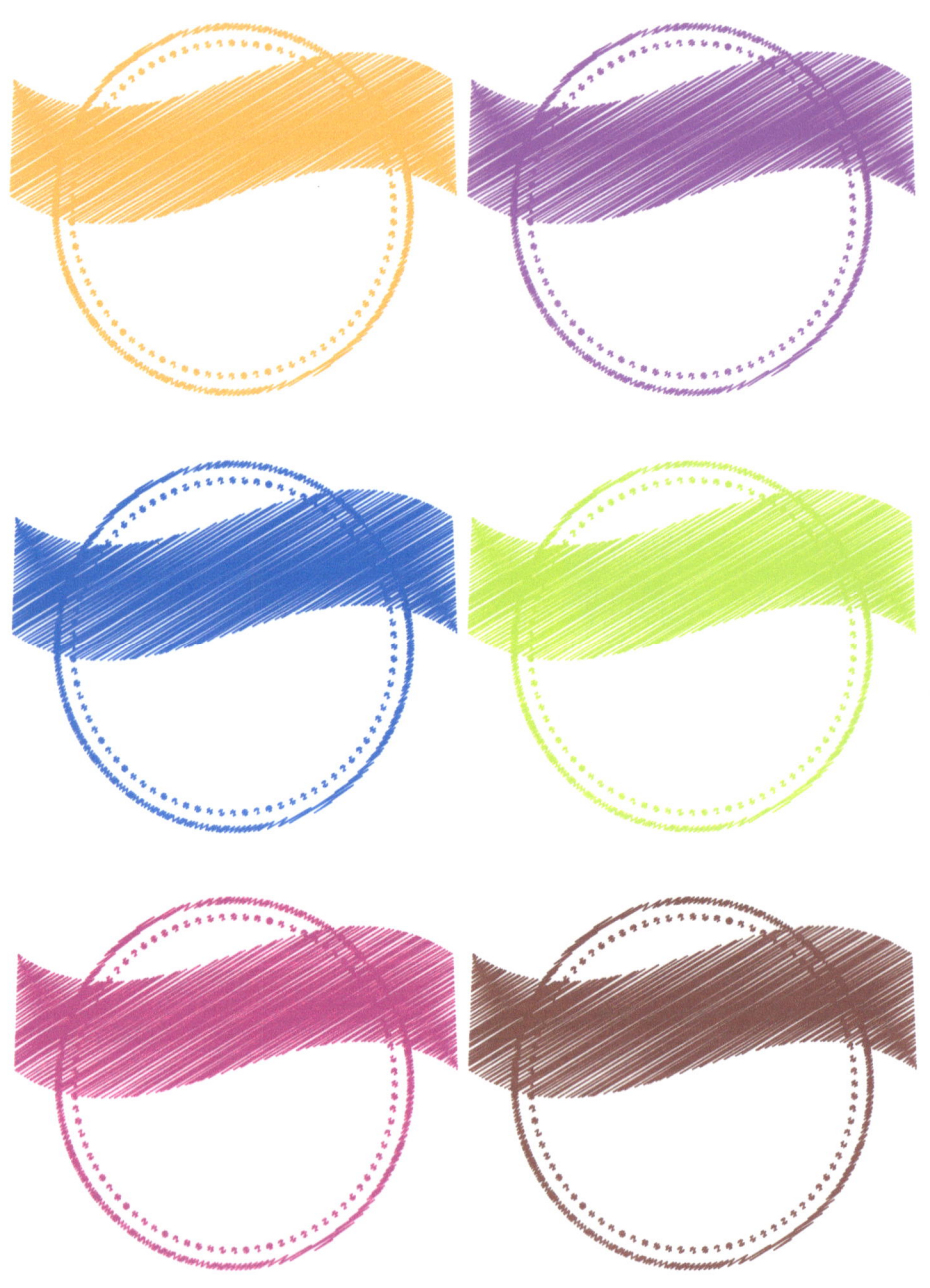

FOOD TRACKER

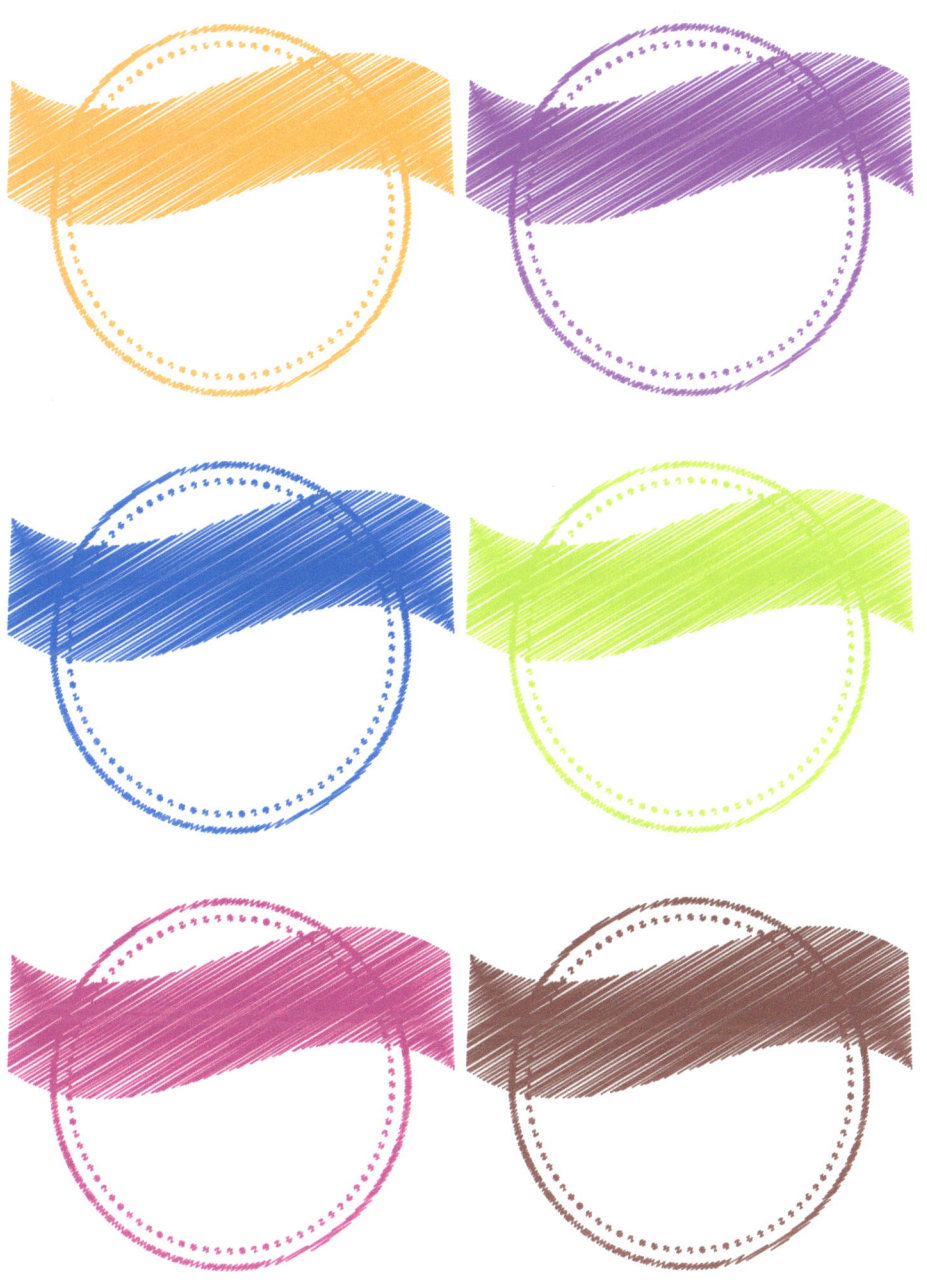

FOOD TRACKER

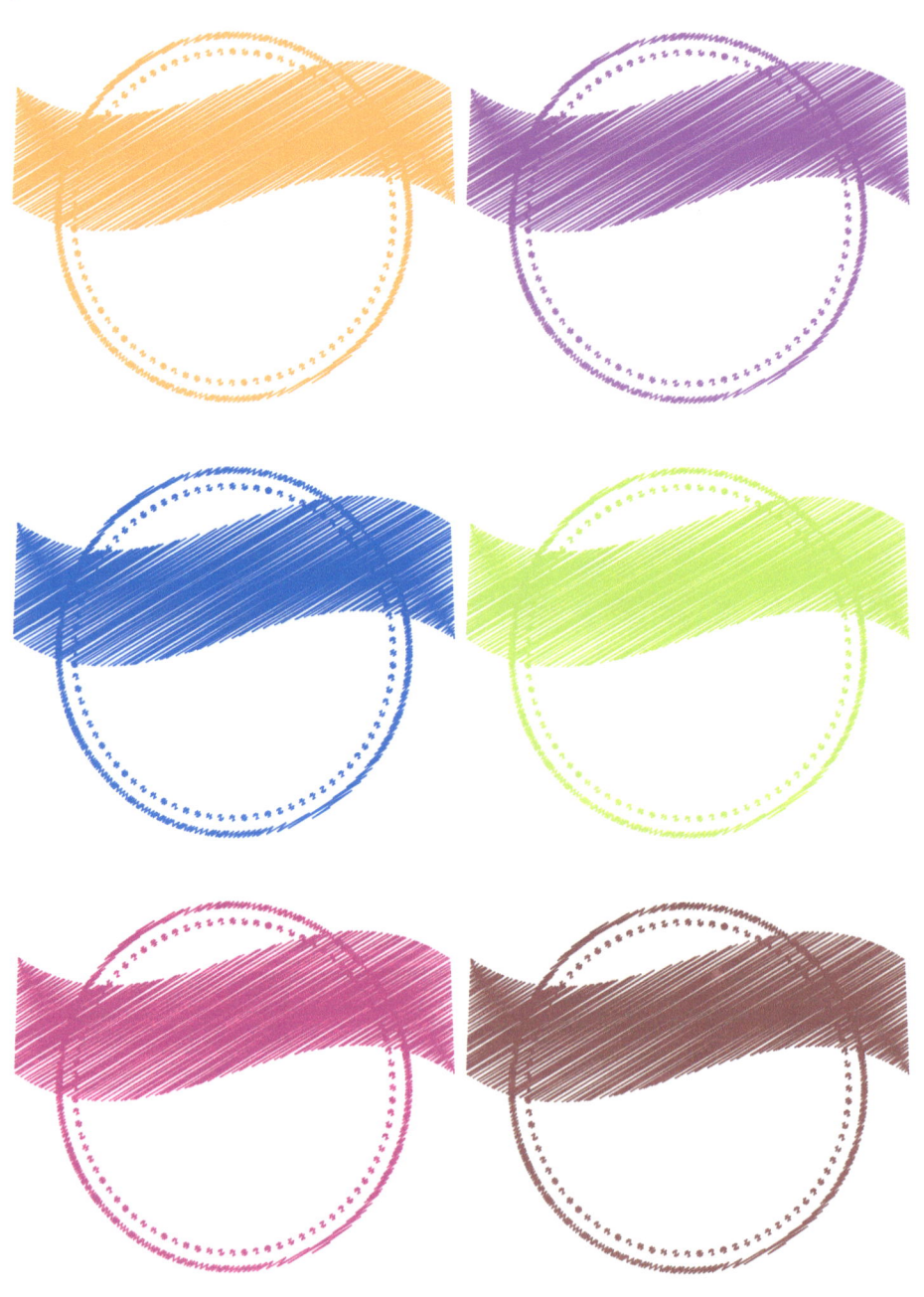

FOOD TRACKER

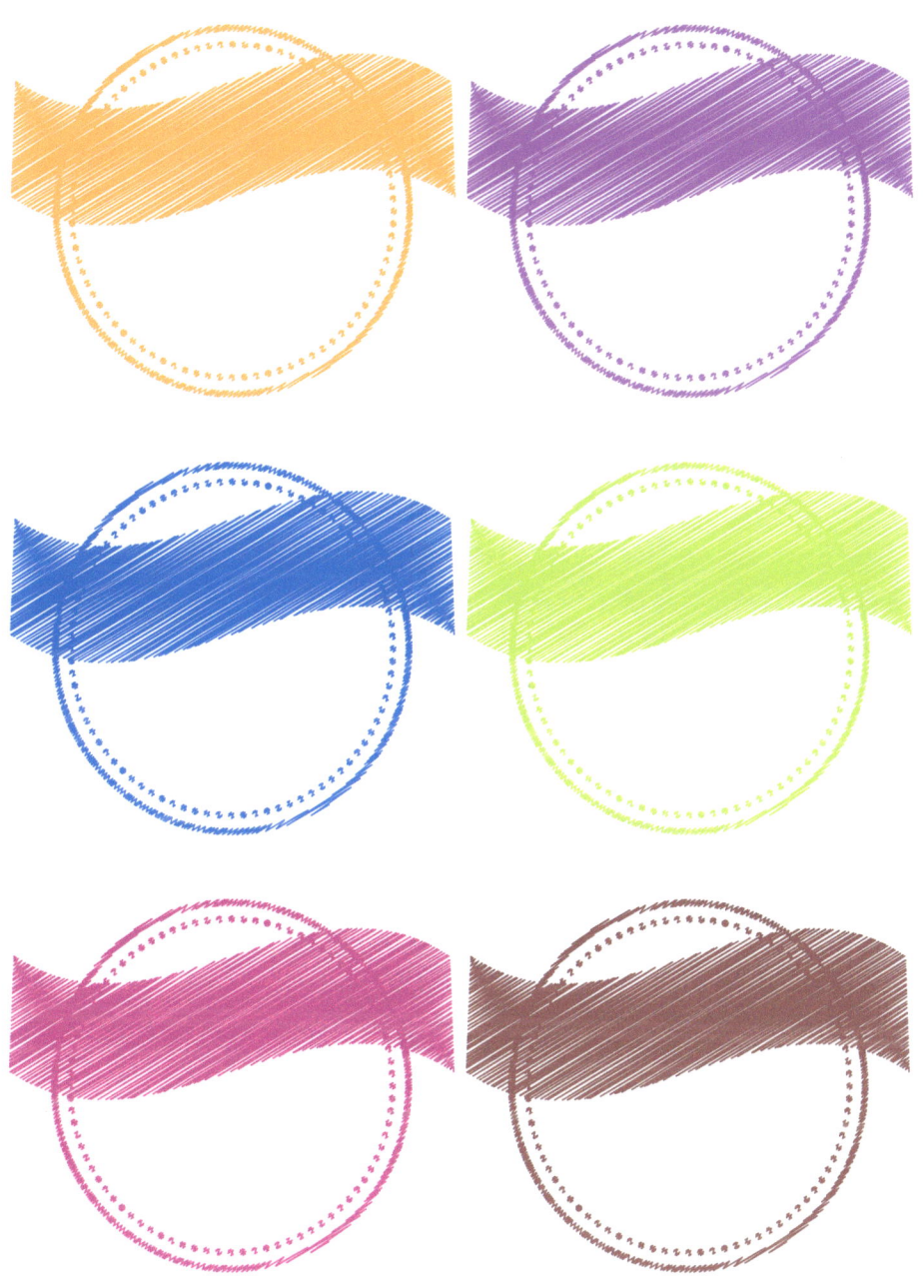

FOOD TRACKER

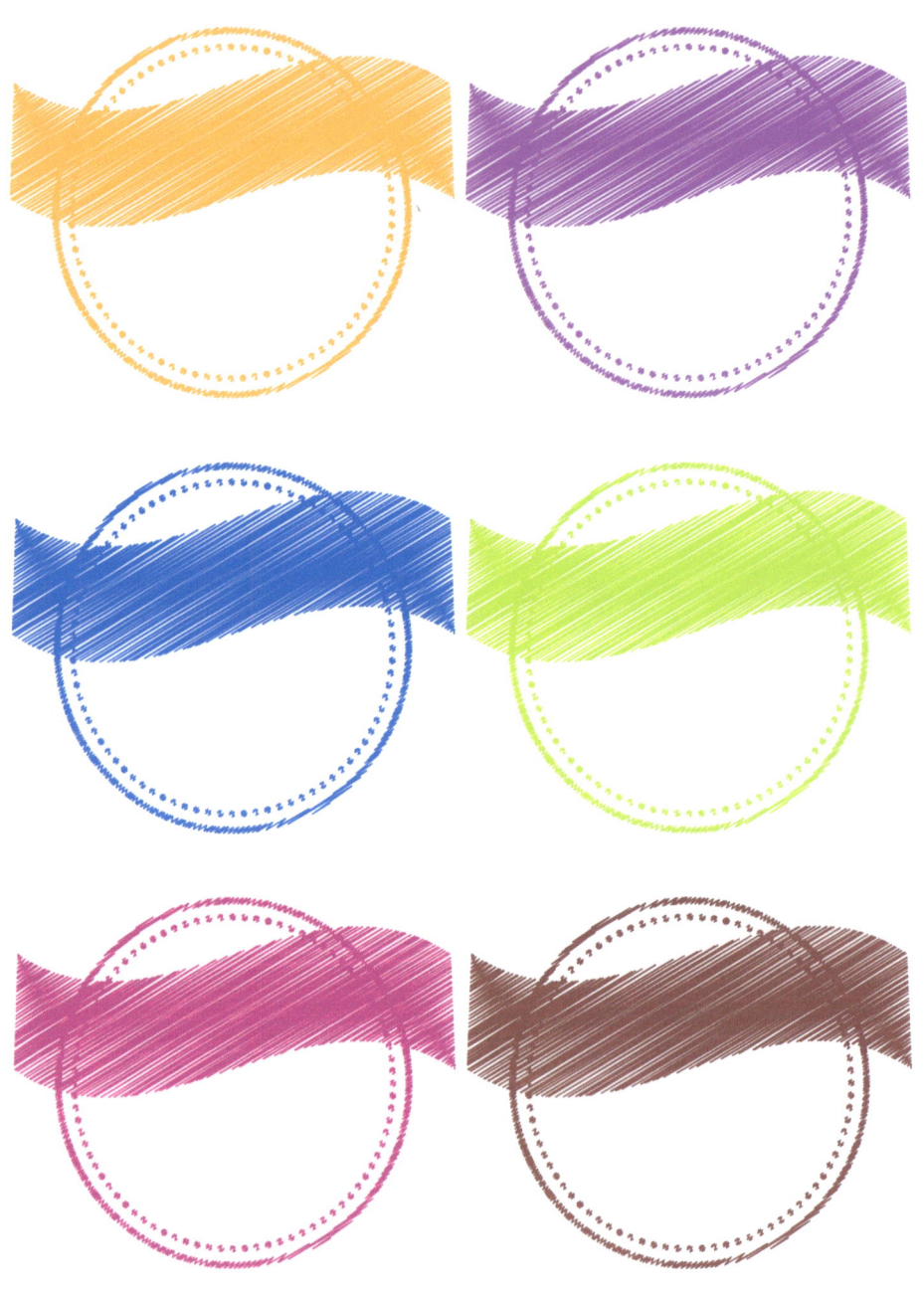

FOOD TRACKER

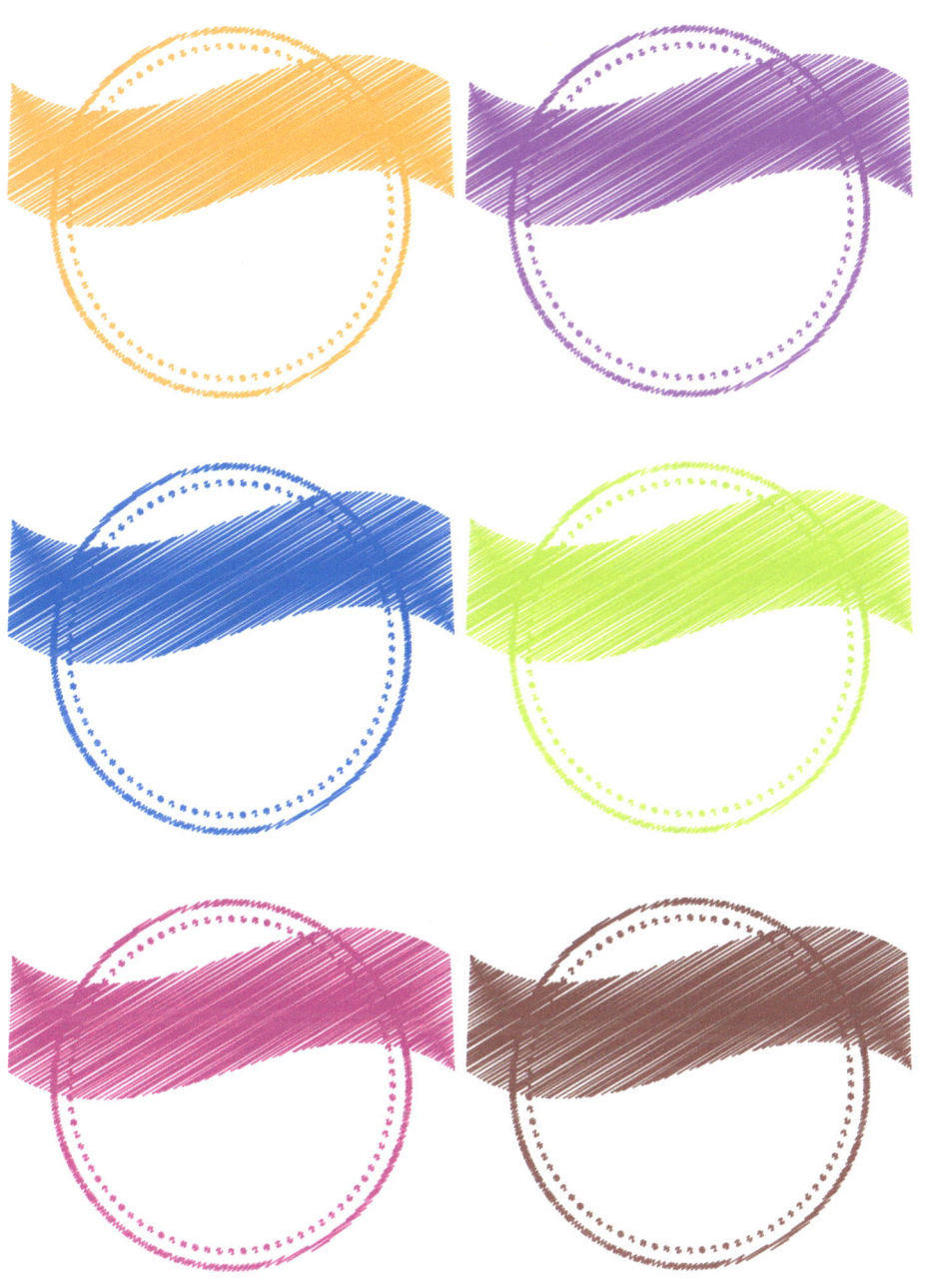

FOOD TRACKER

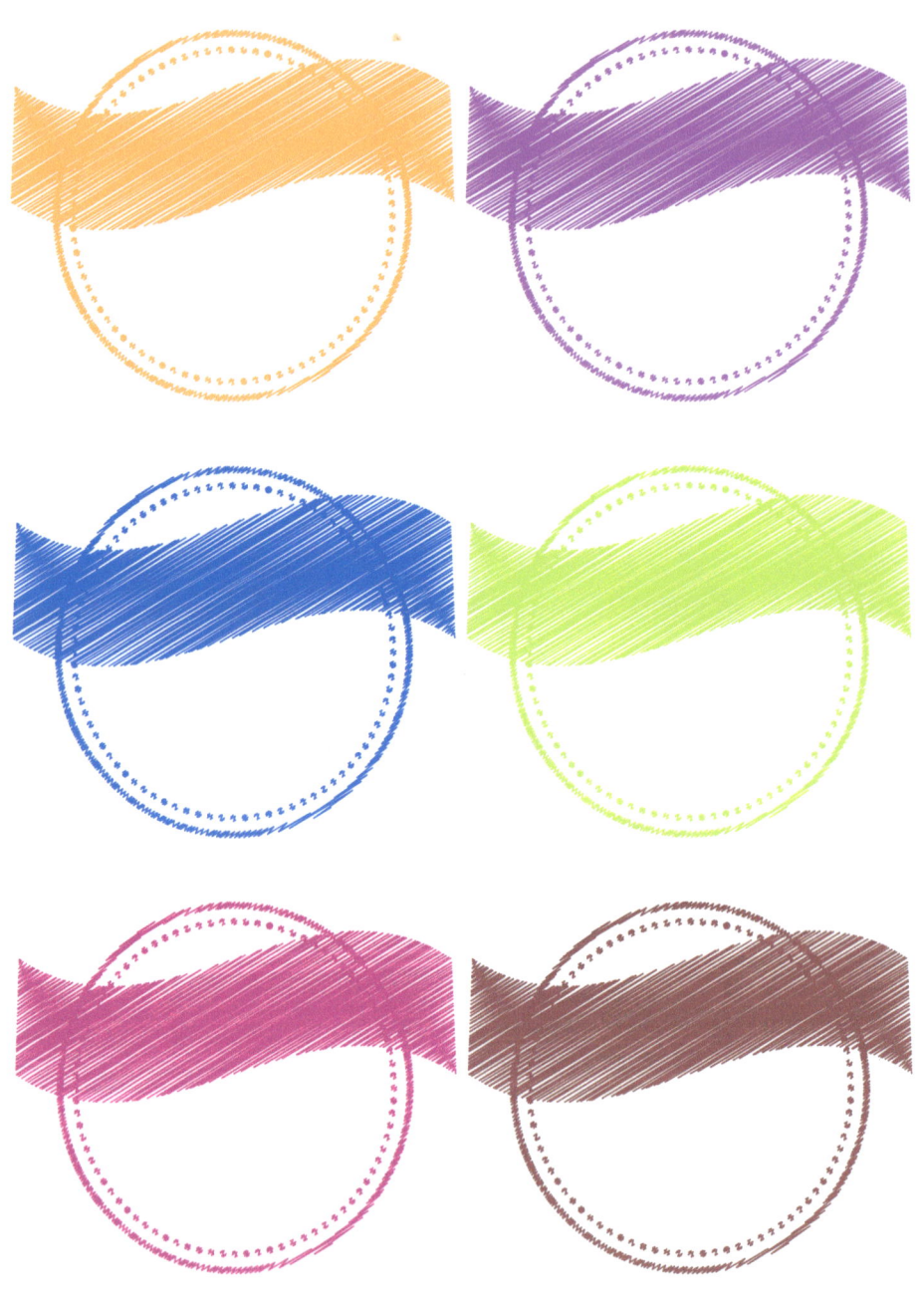

FOOD TRACKER

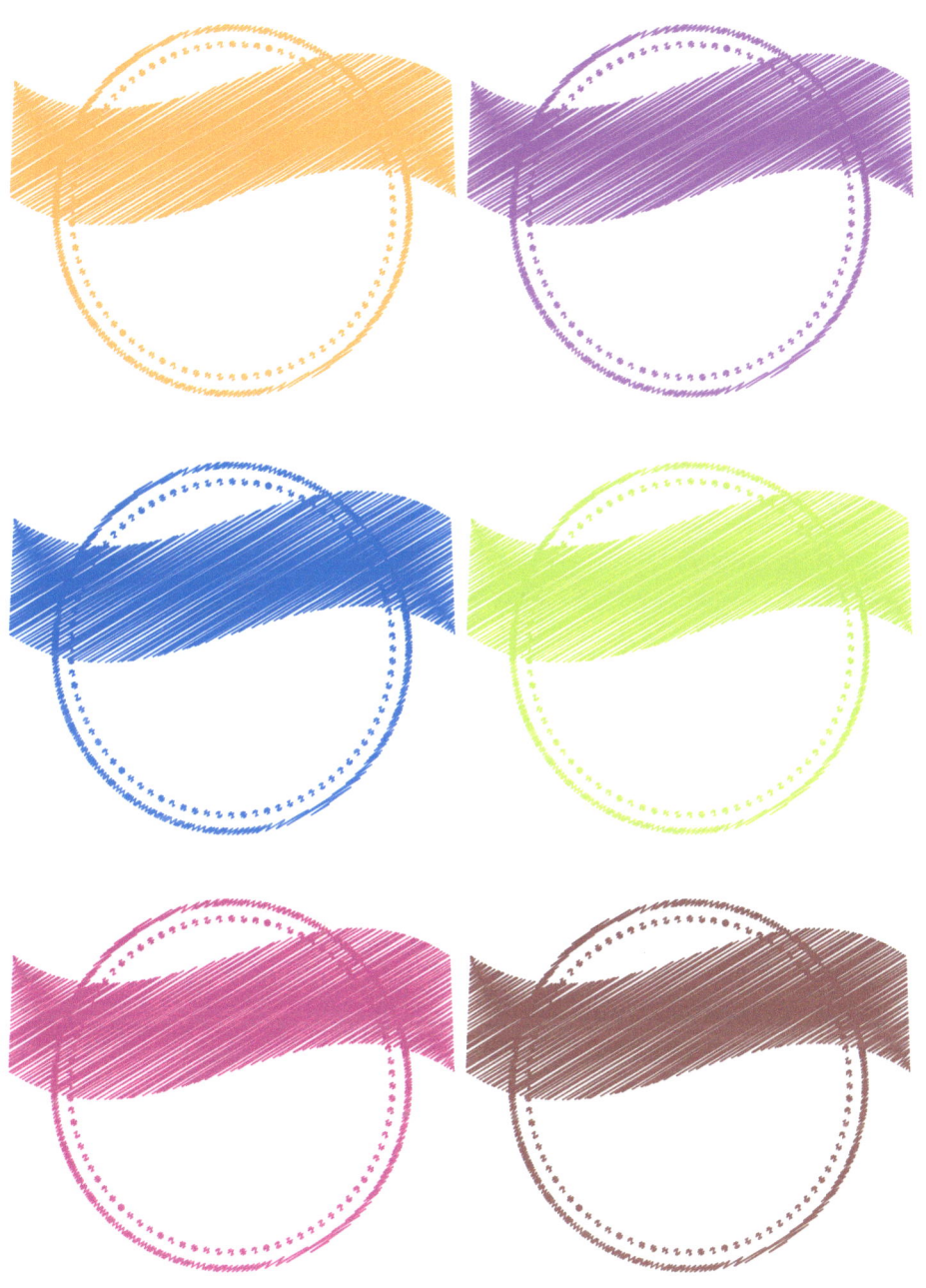

FOOD TRACKER

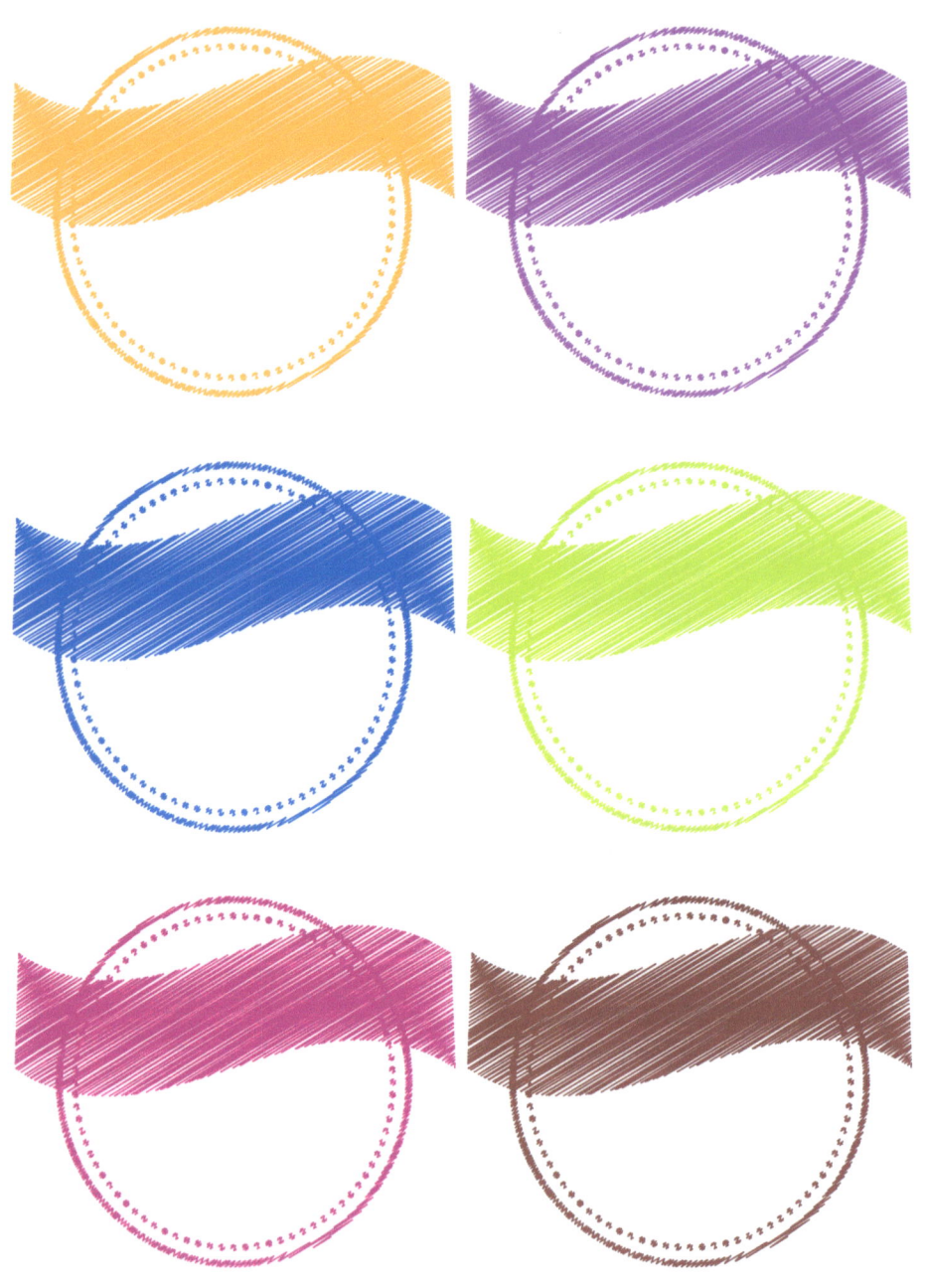

FOOD TRACKER

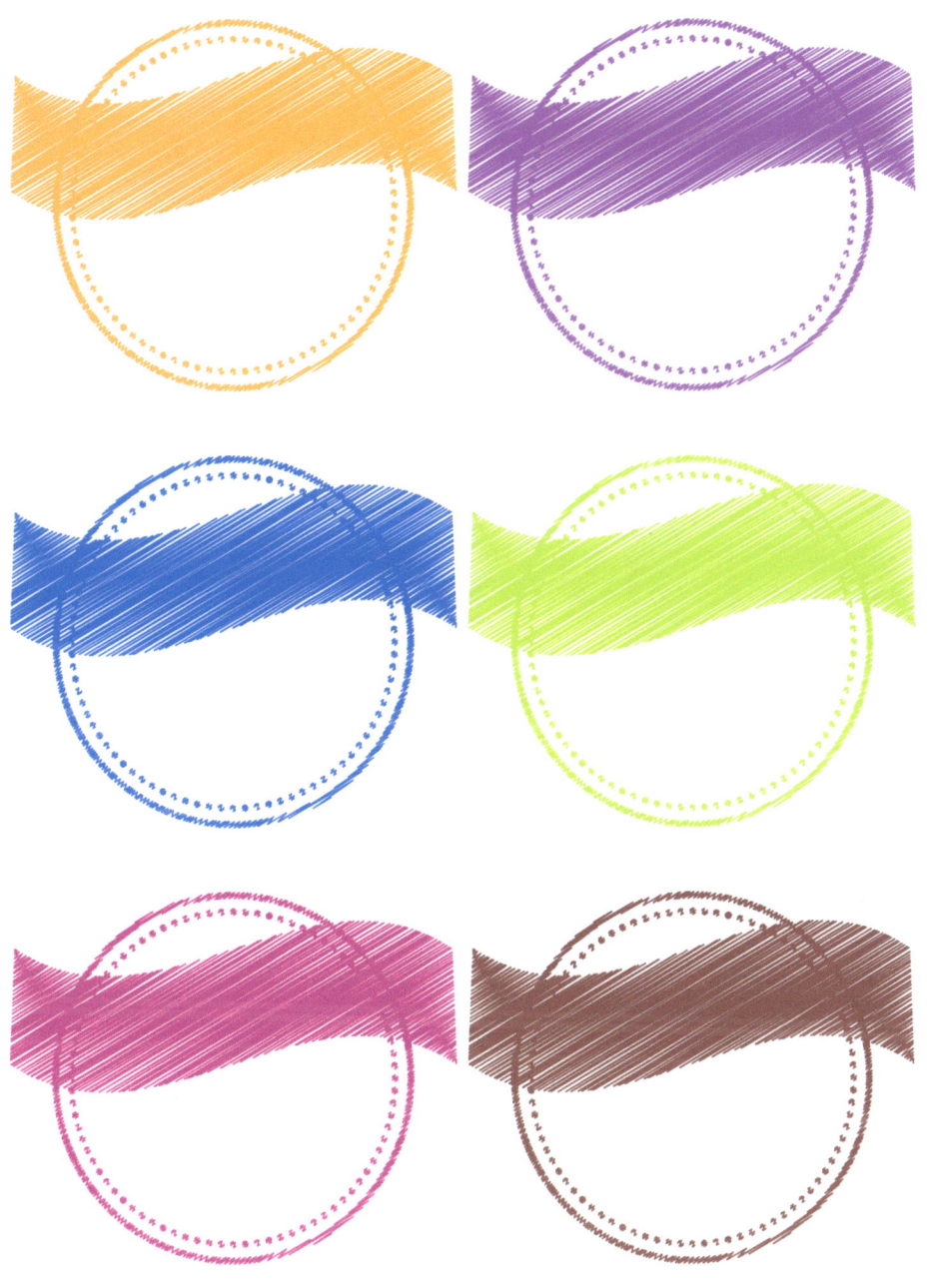

FOOD TRACKER

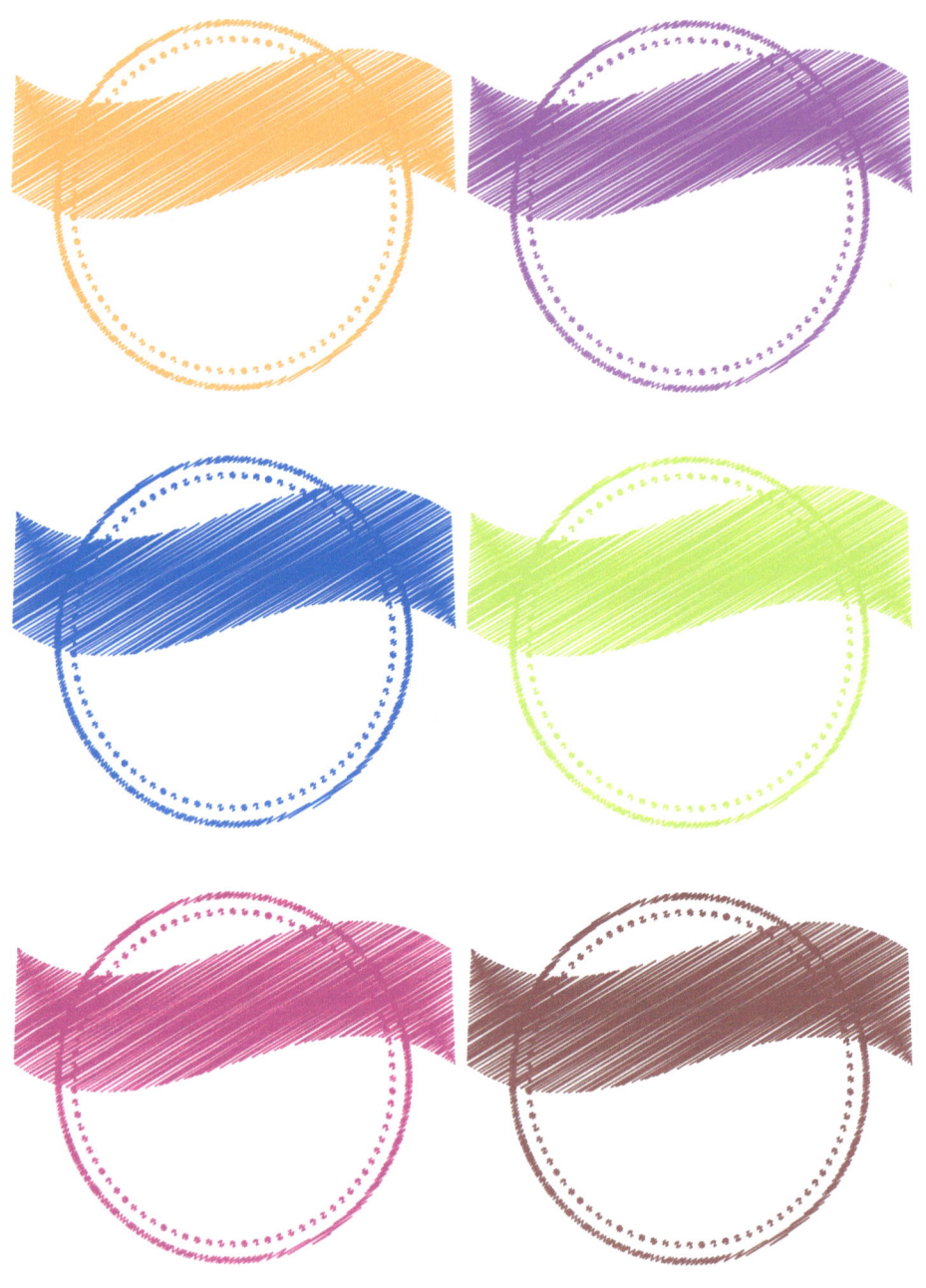

FOOD TRACKER

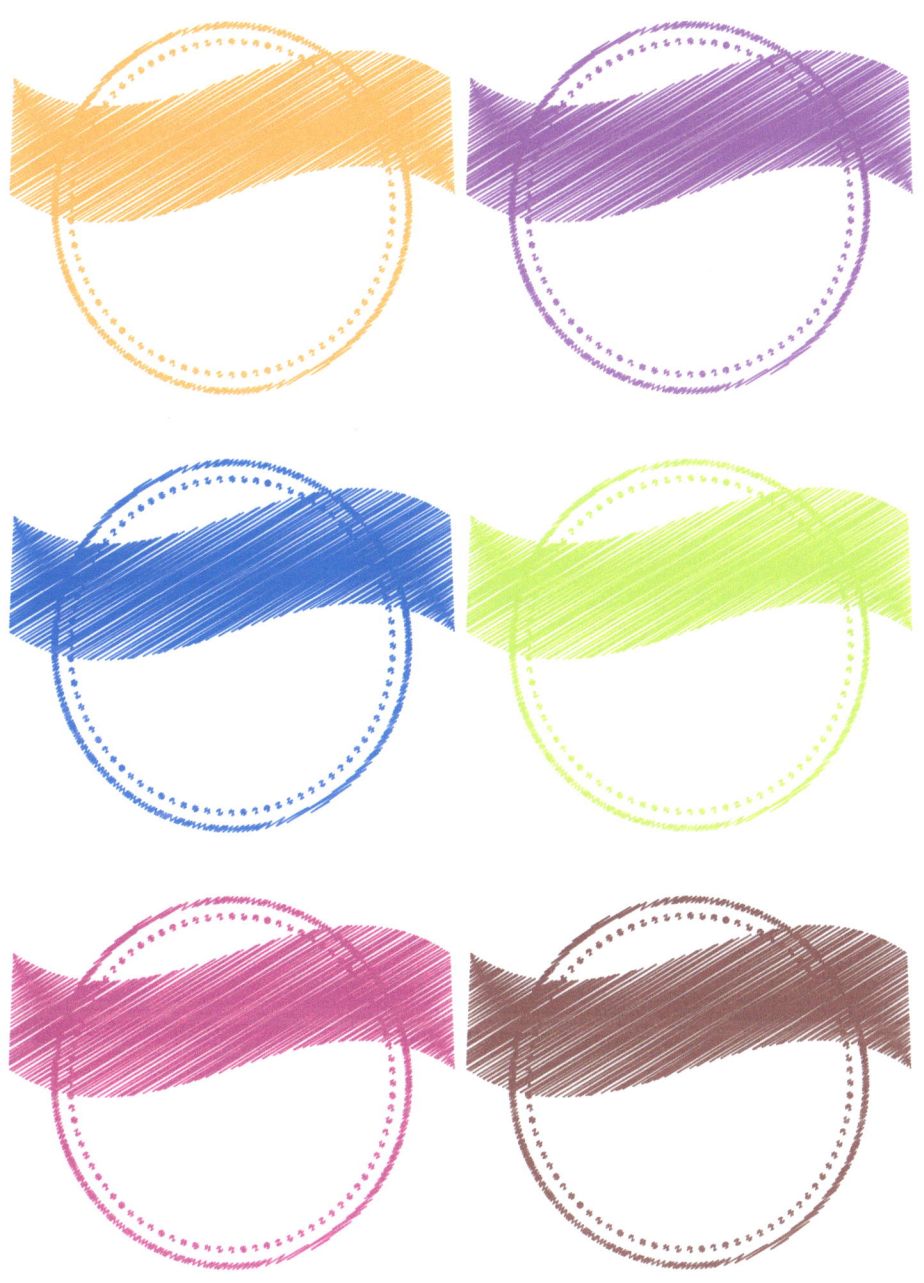

FOOD TRACKER

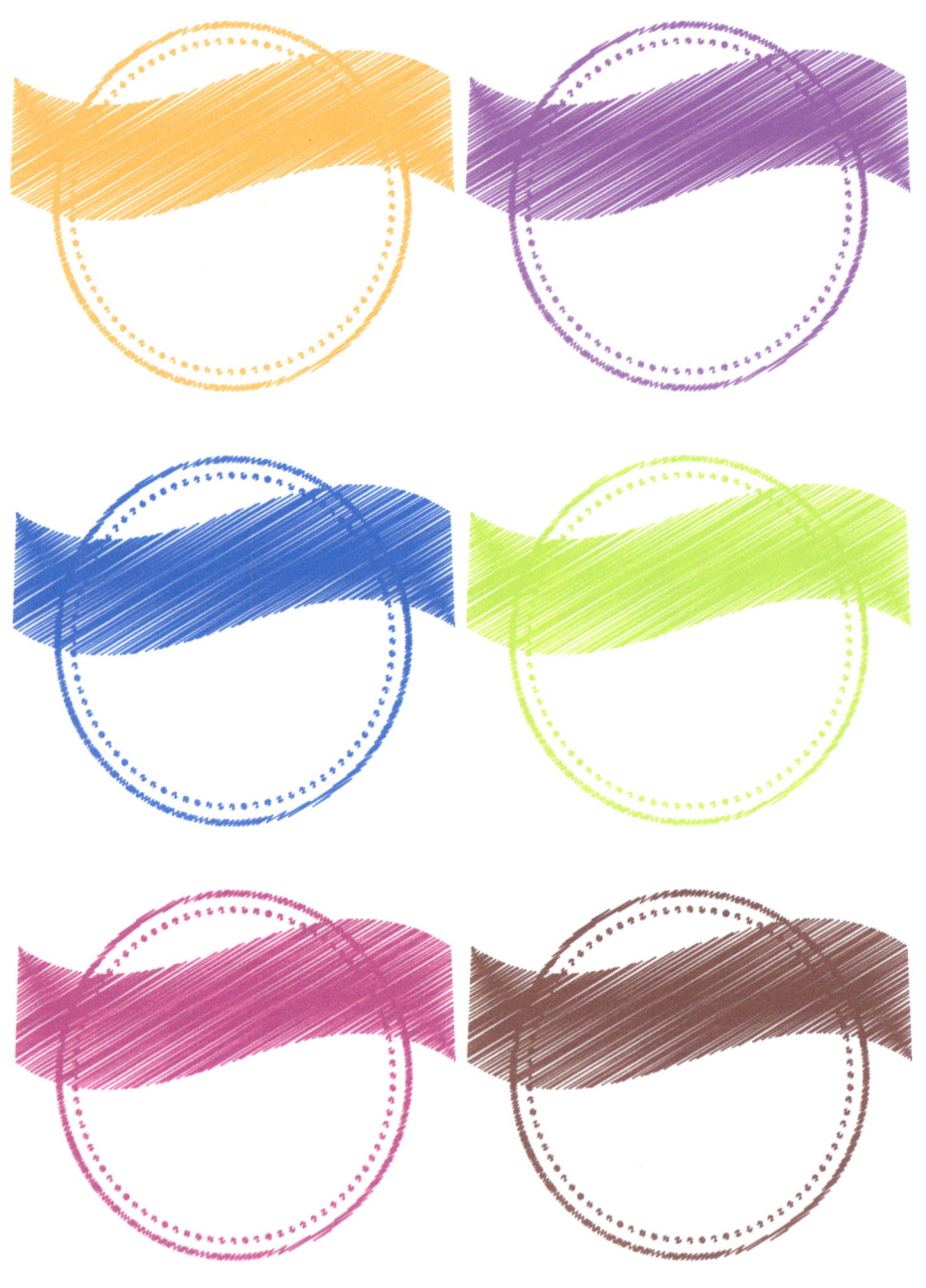

FOOD TRACKER

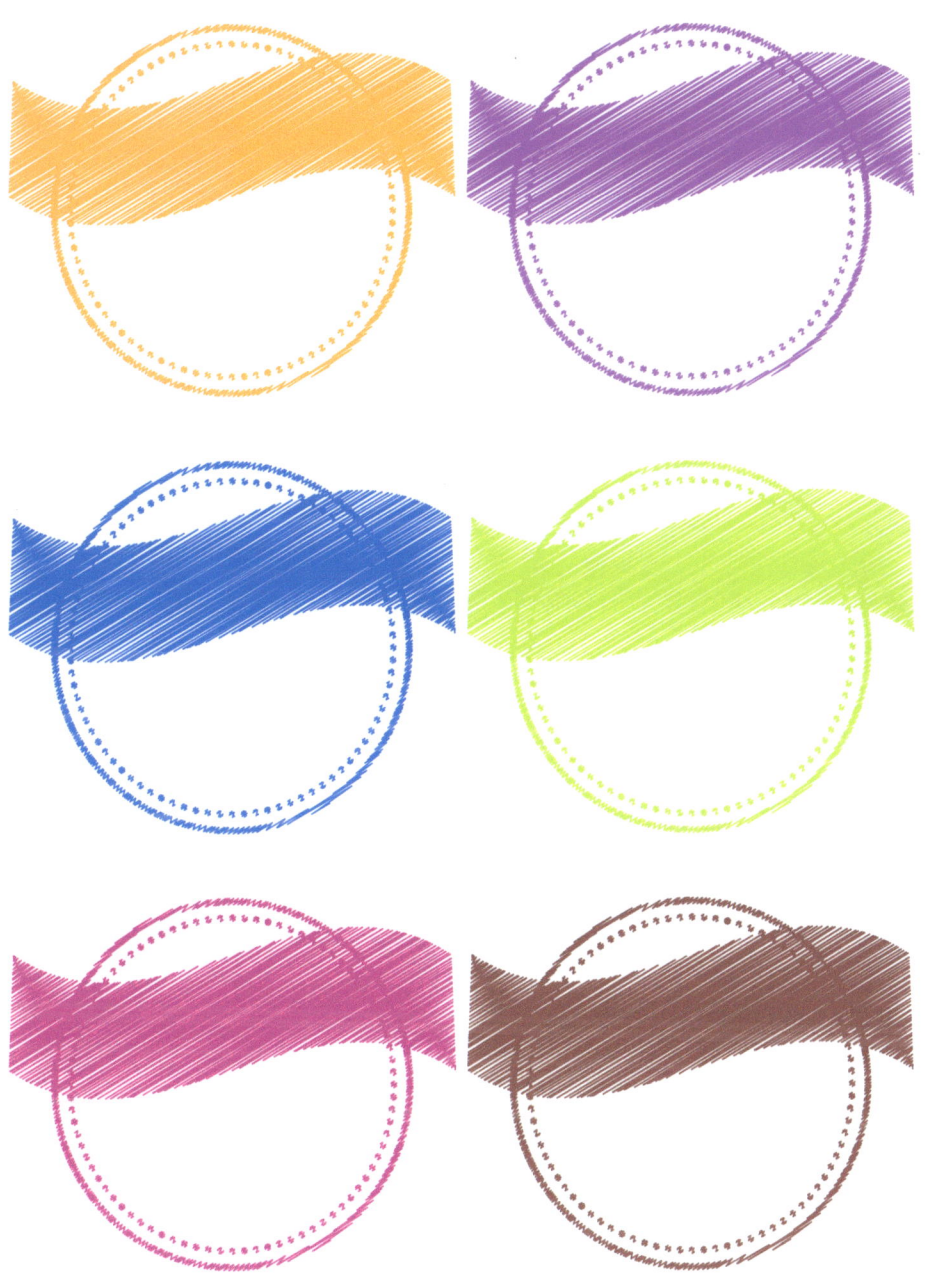

FOOD TRACKER

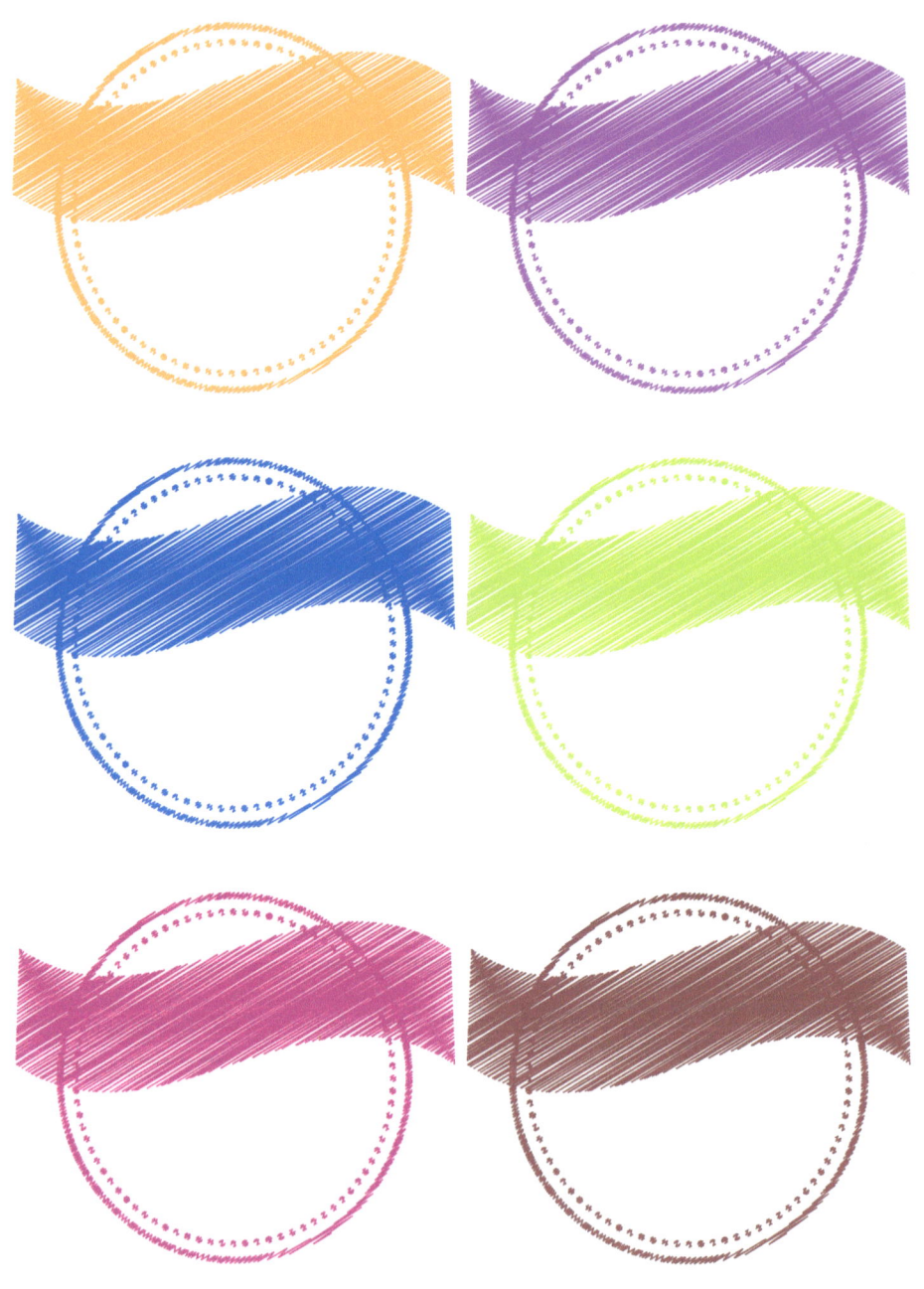

FOOD TRACKER

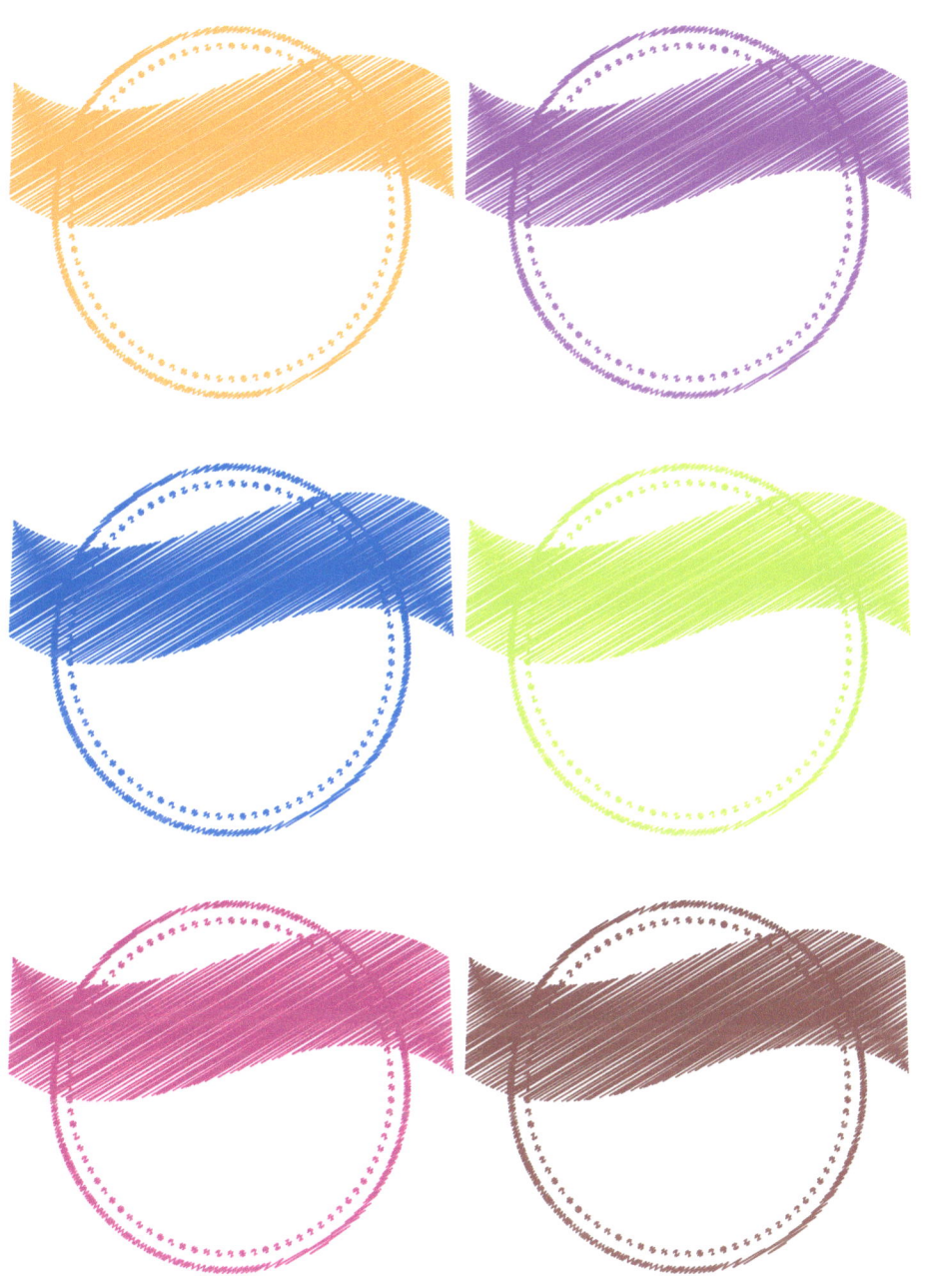

FOOD TRACKER

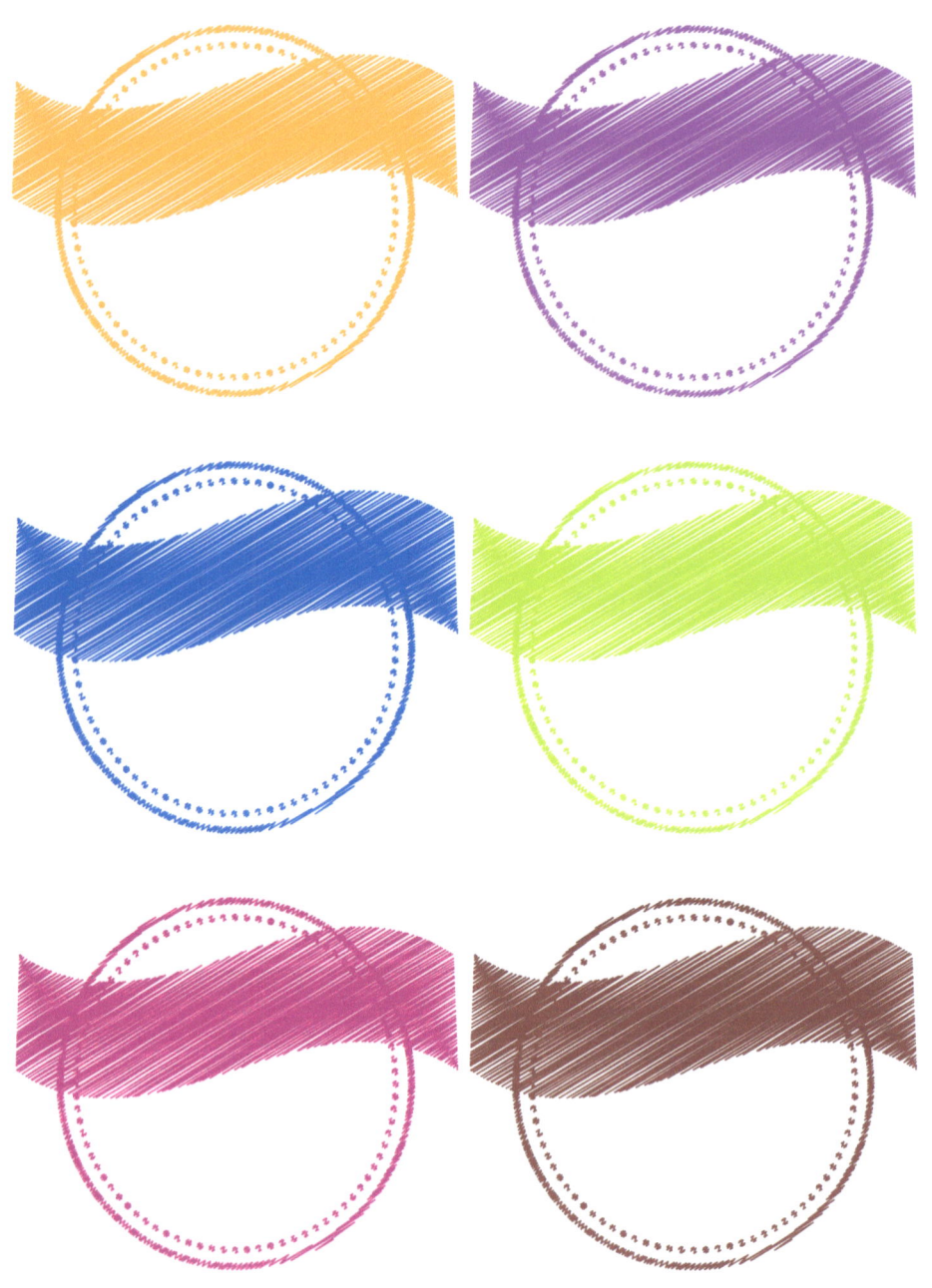

FOOD TRACKER

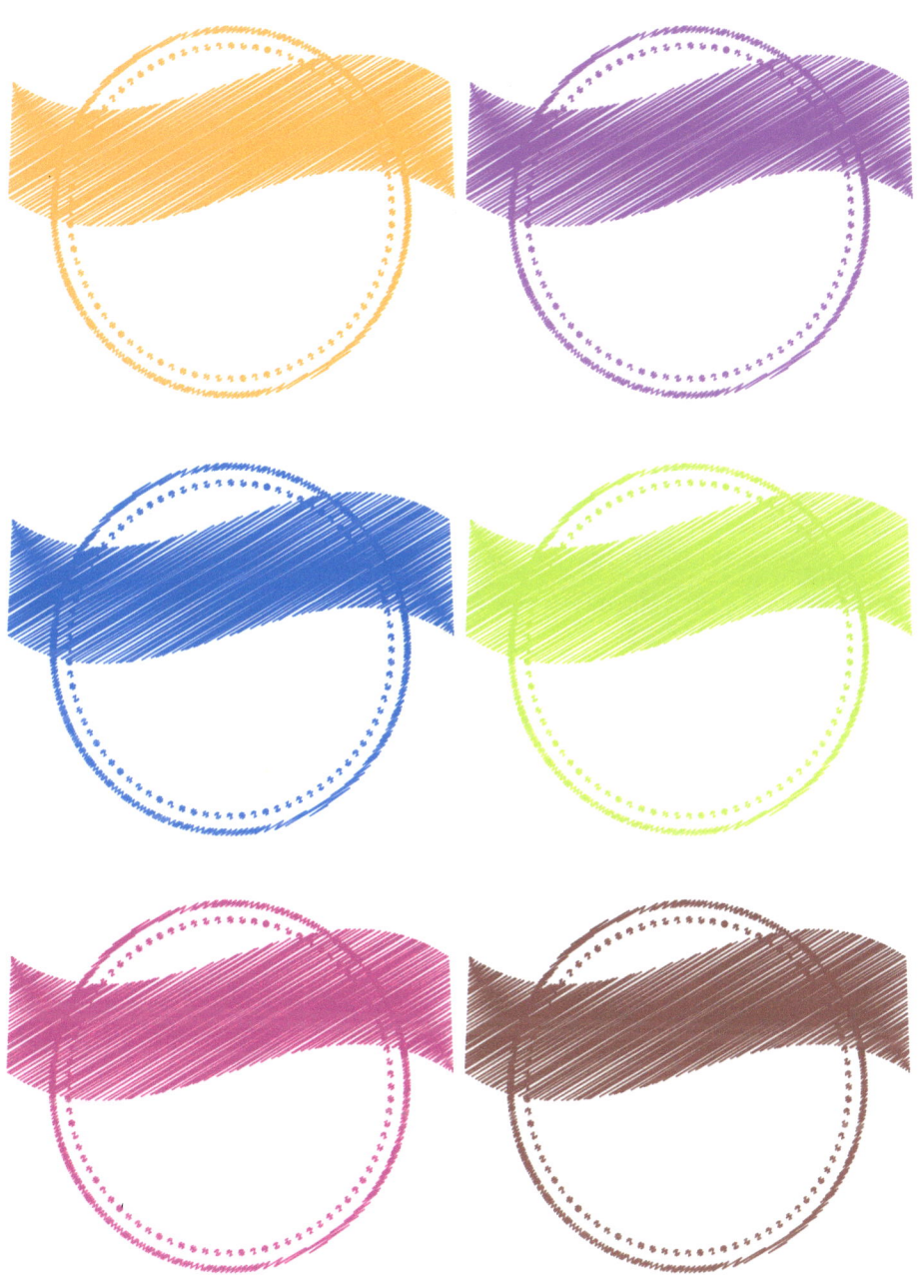

FOOD TRACKER

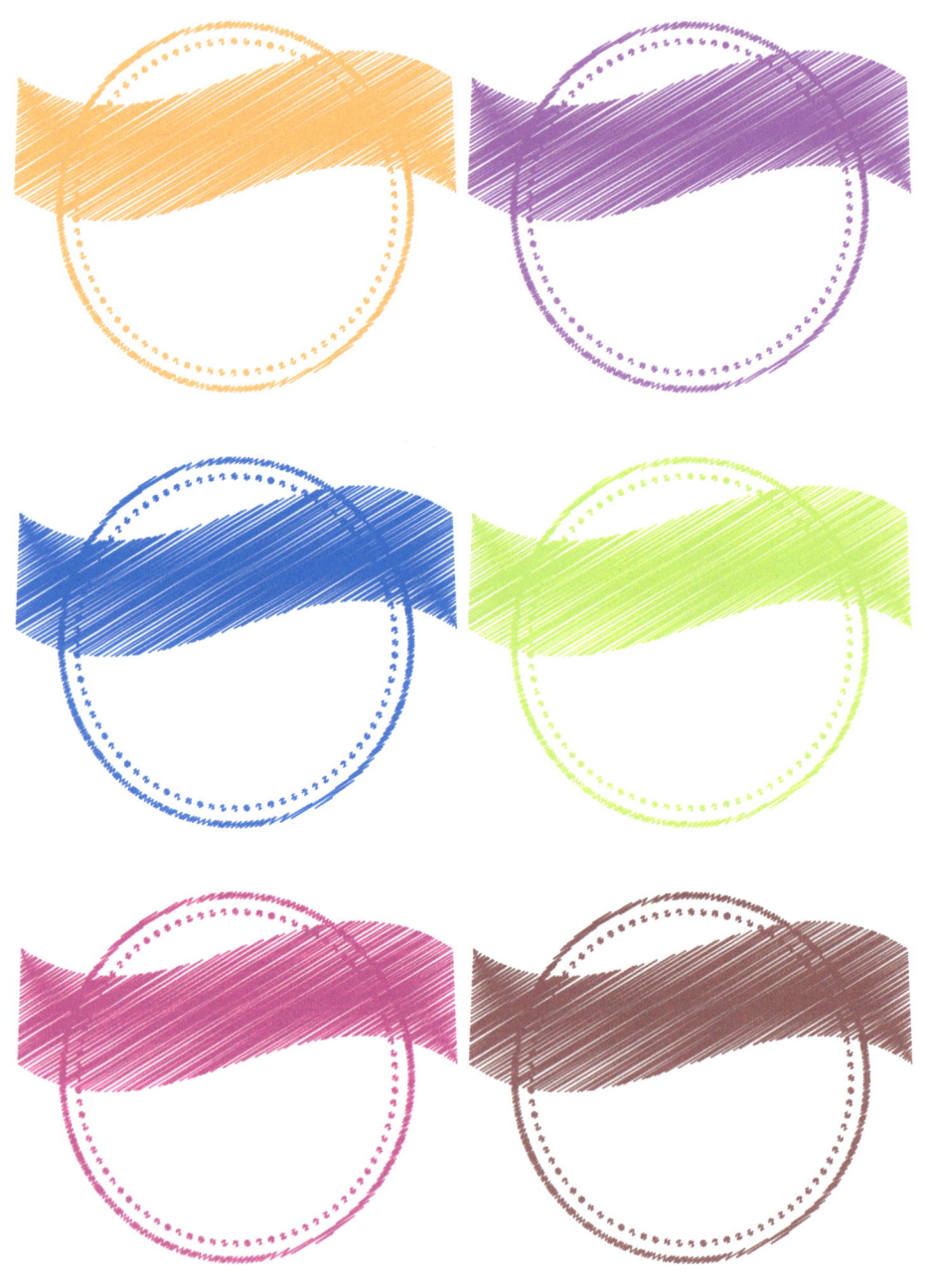

FOOD TRACKER

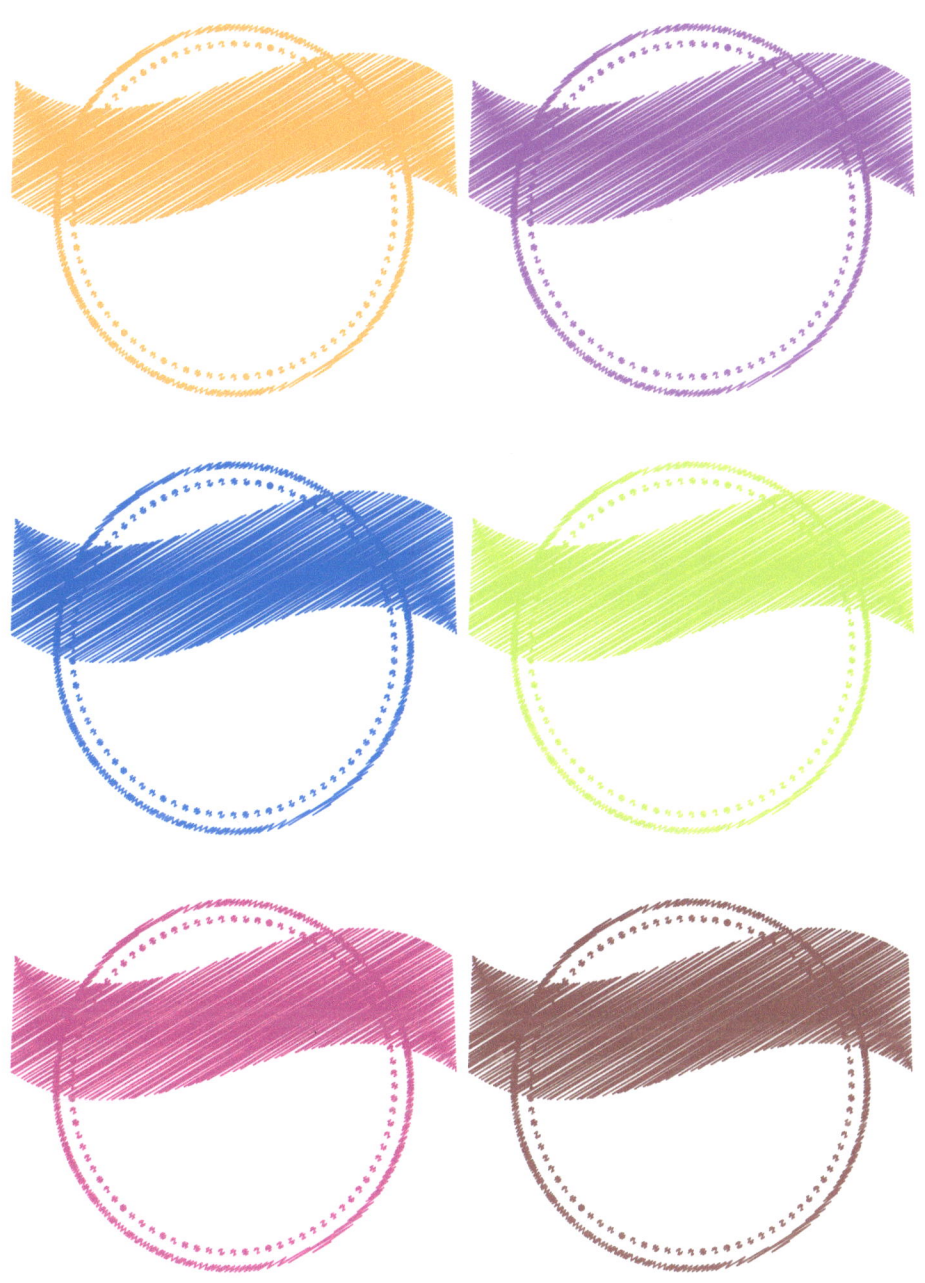

FOOD TRACKER

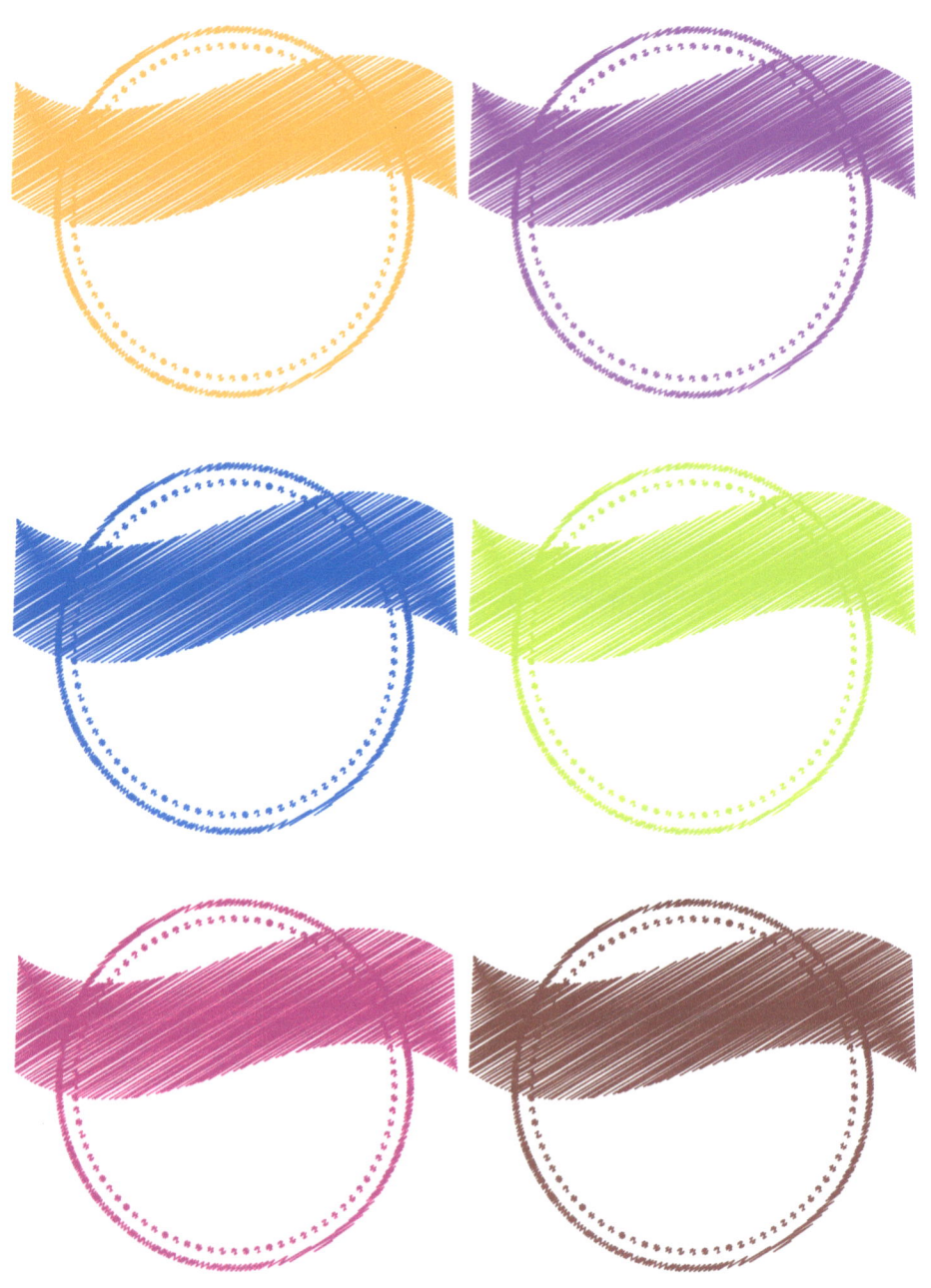

FOOD TRACKER

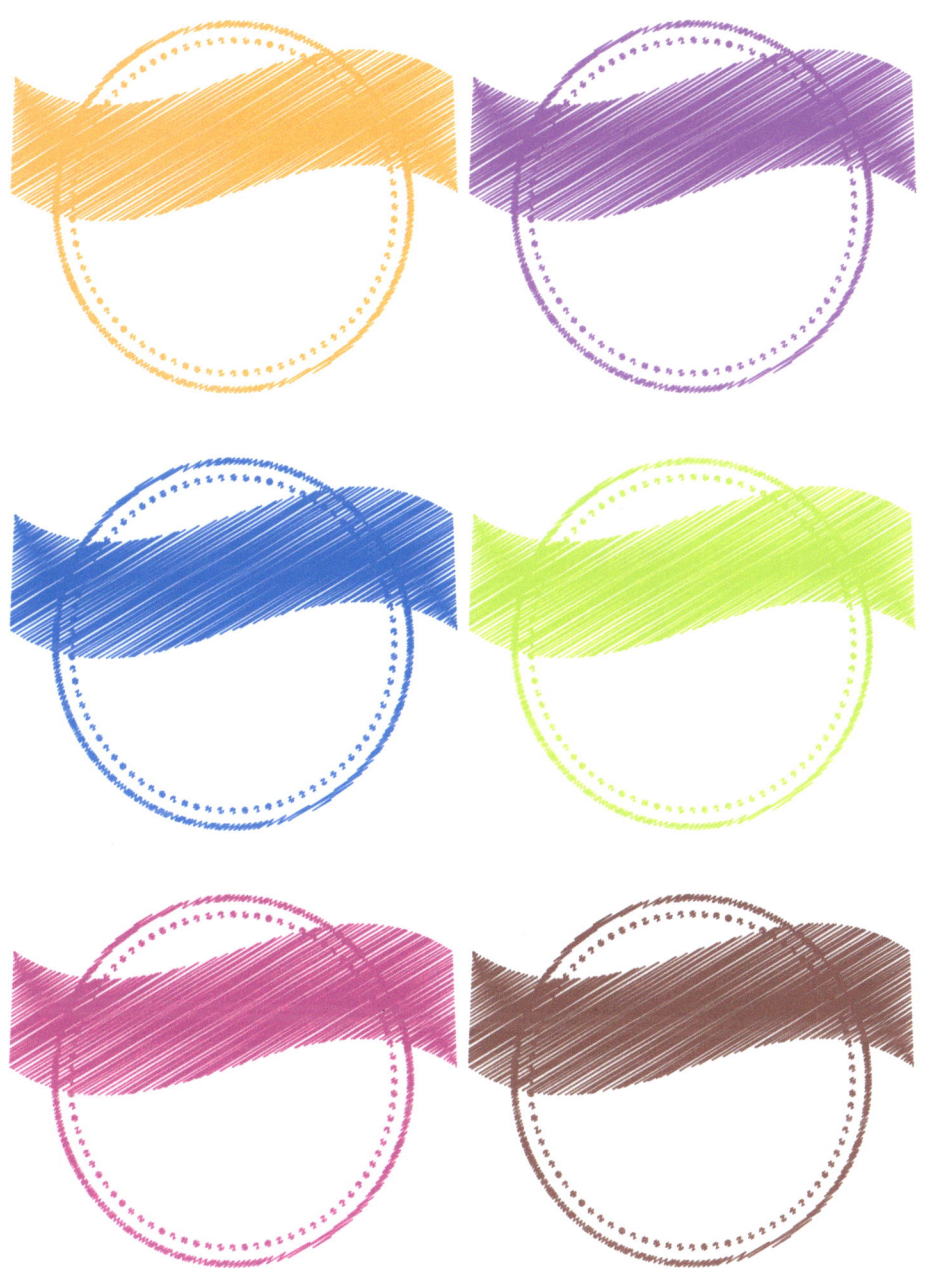

FOOD TRACKER

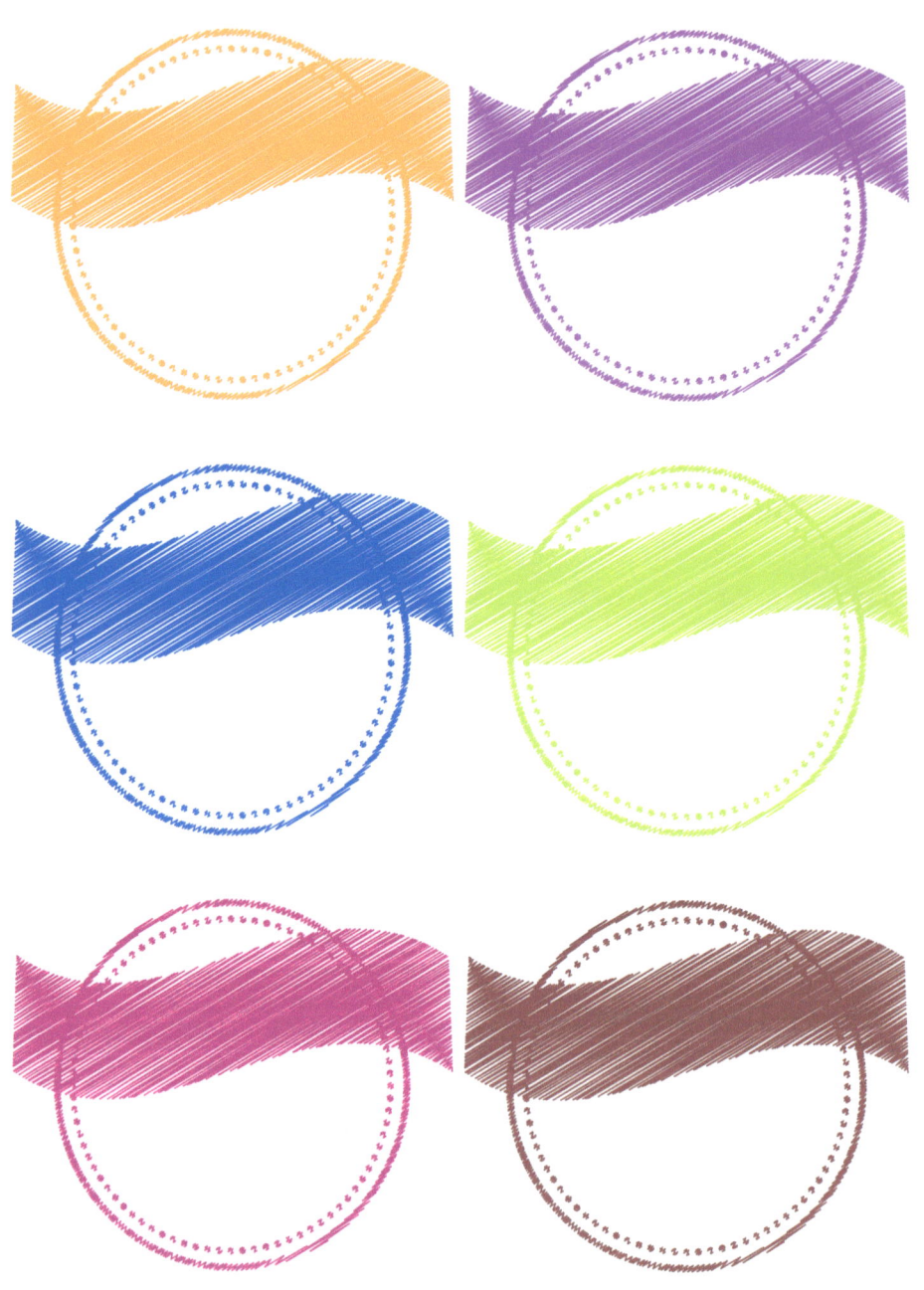

FOOD TRACKER

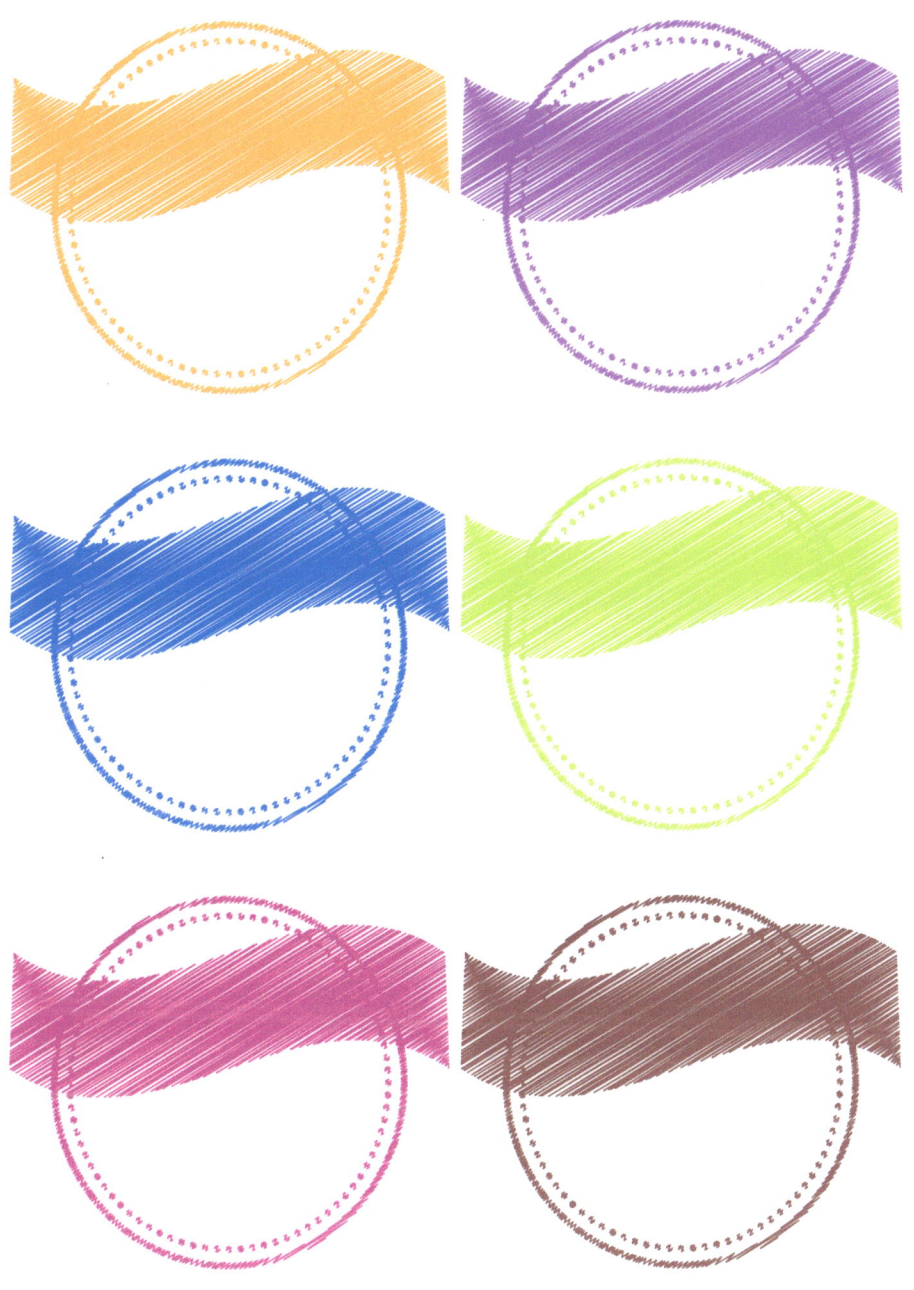

FOOD TRACKER

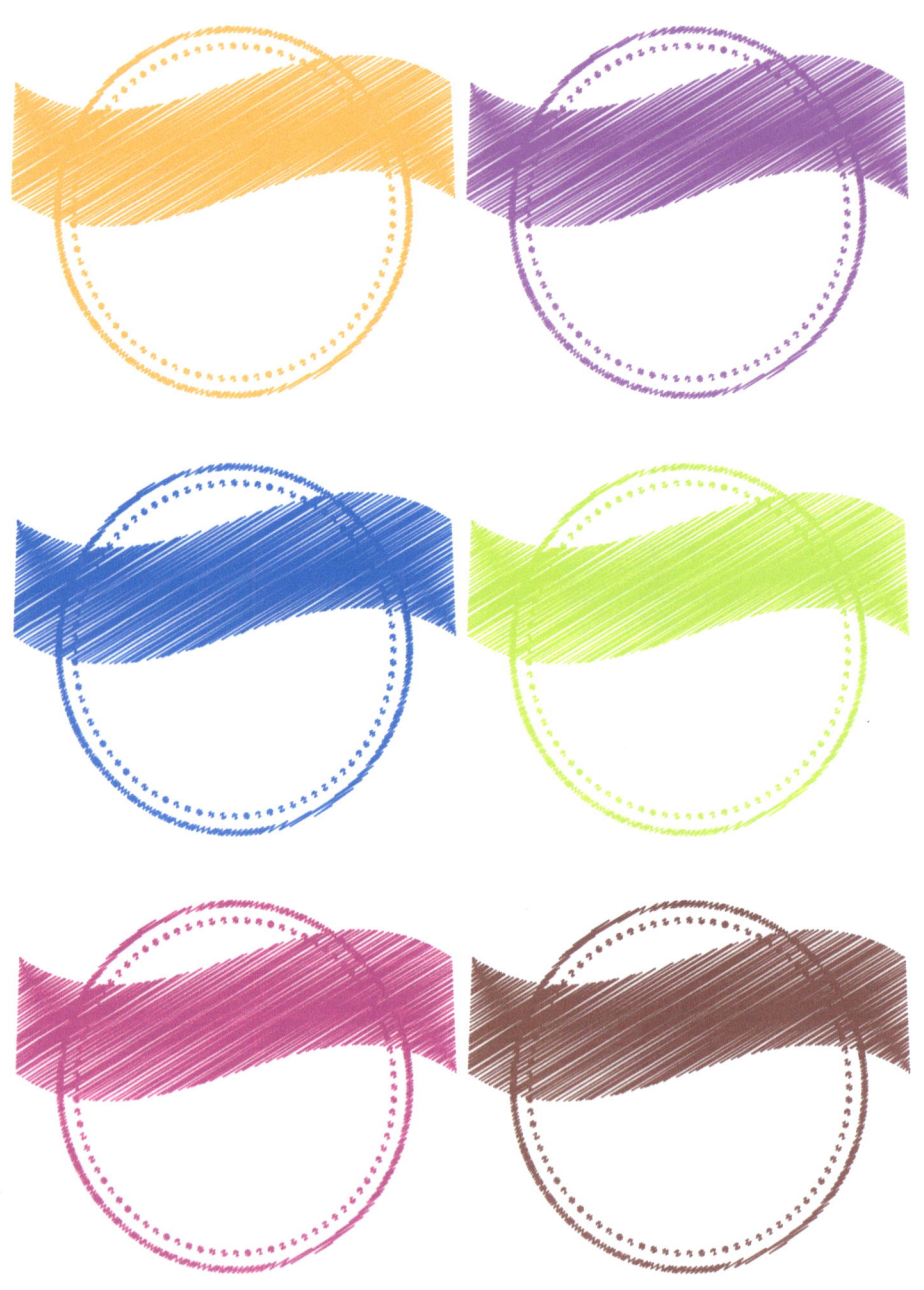

FOOD TRACKER

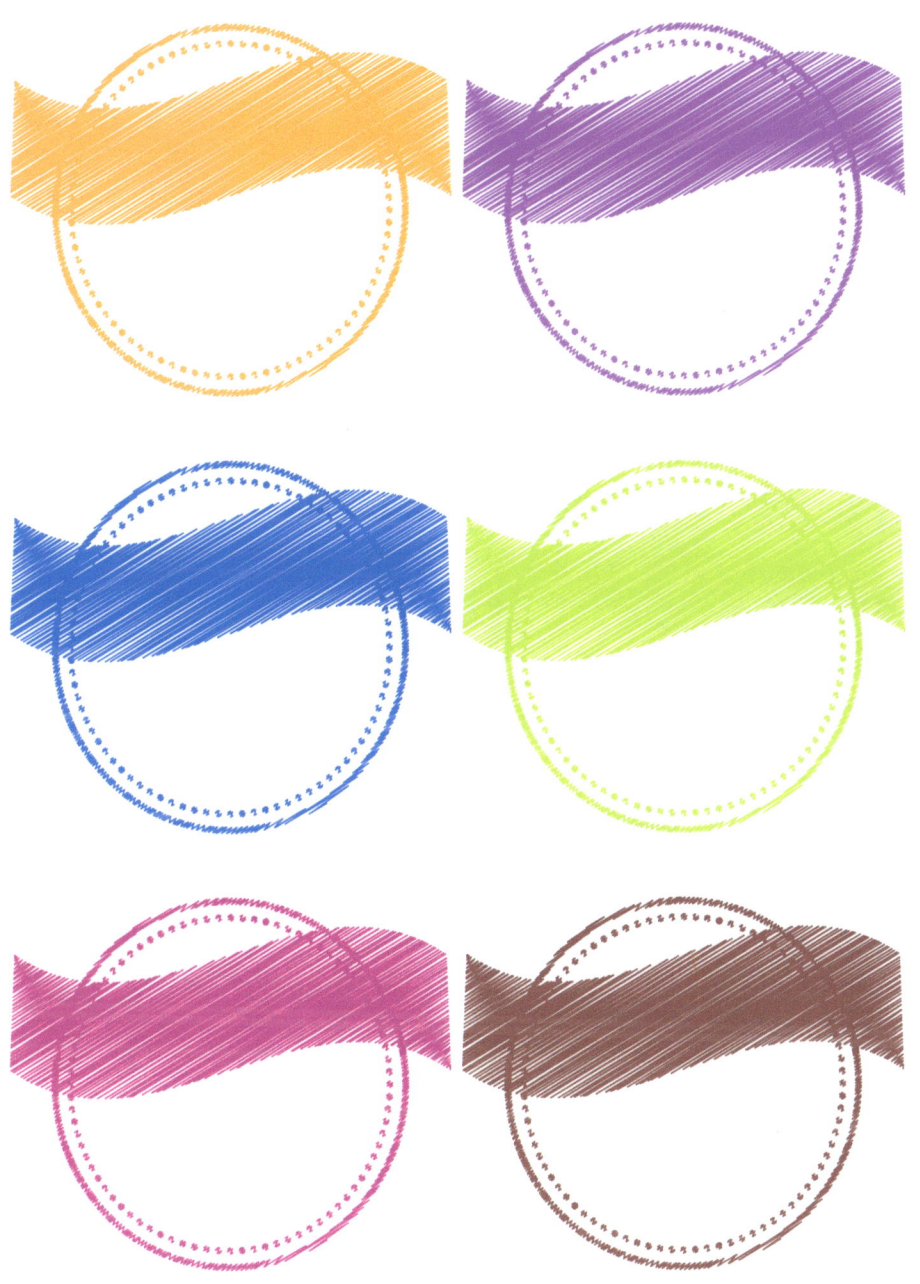

FOOD TRACKER

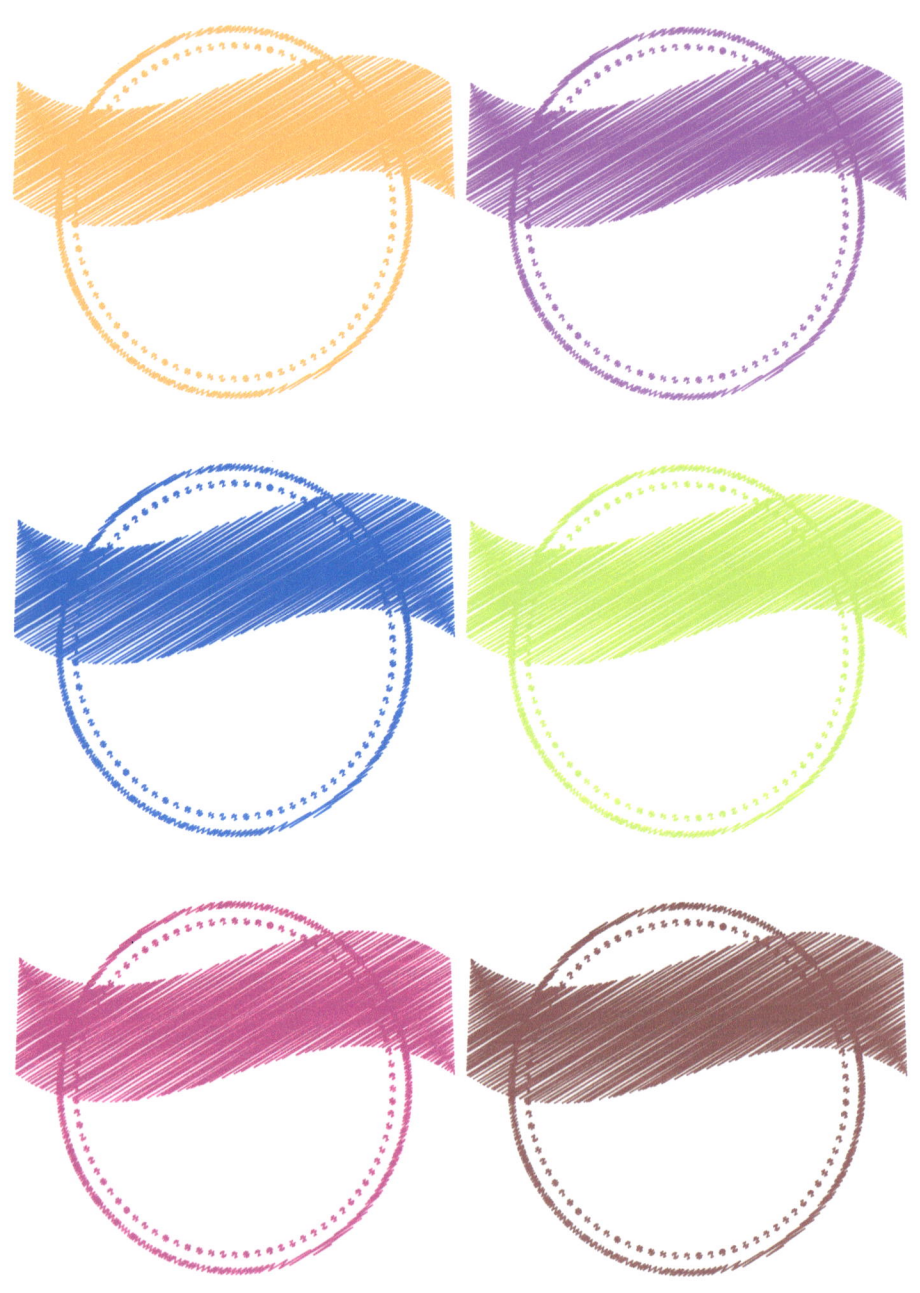

FOOD TRACKER

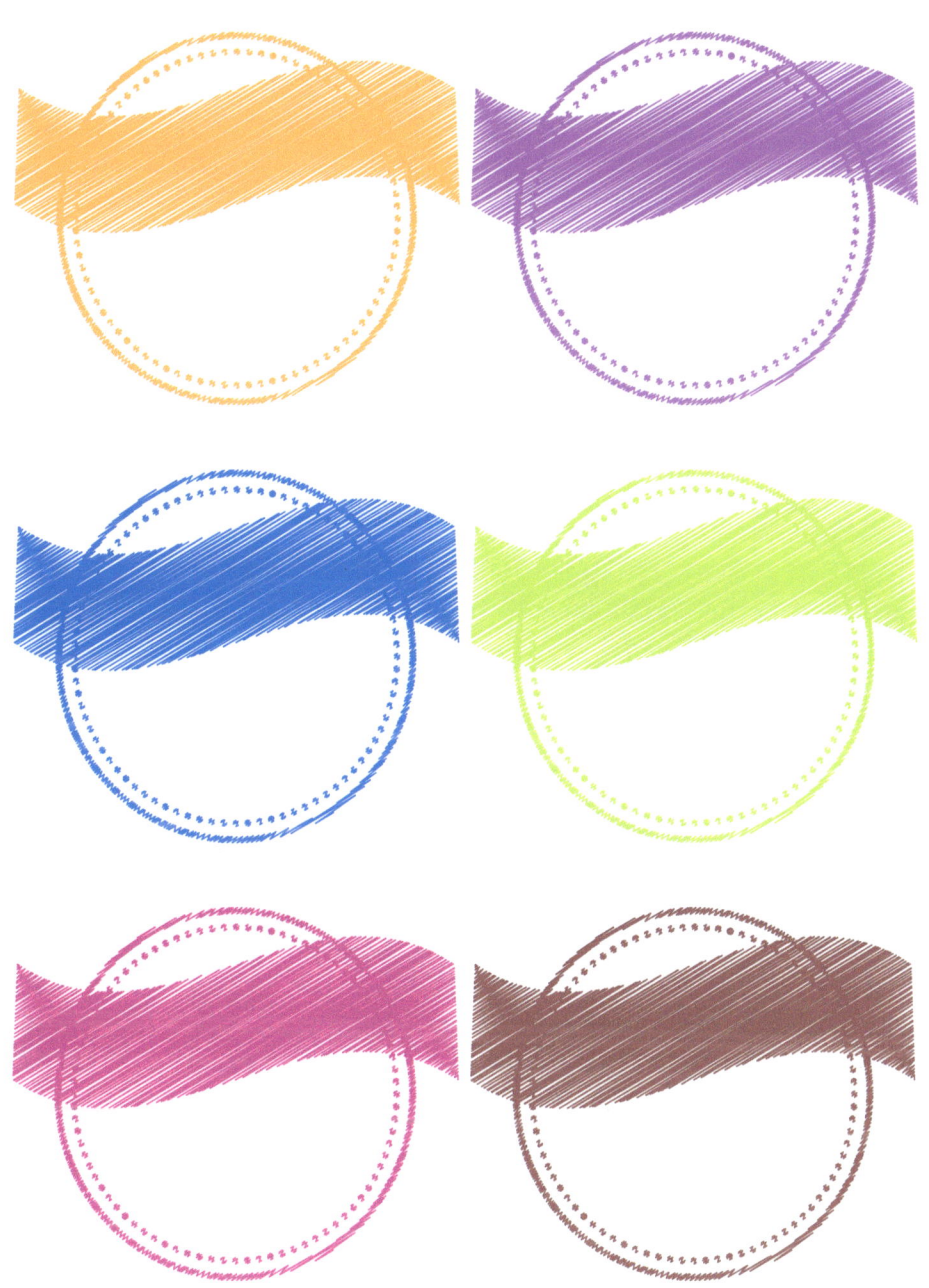

FOOD TRACKER

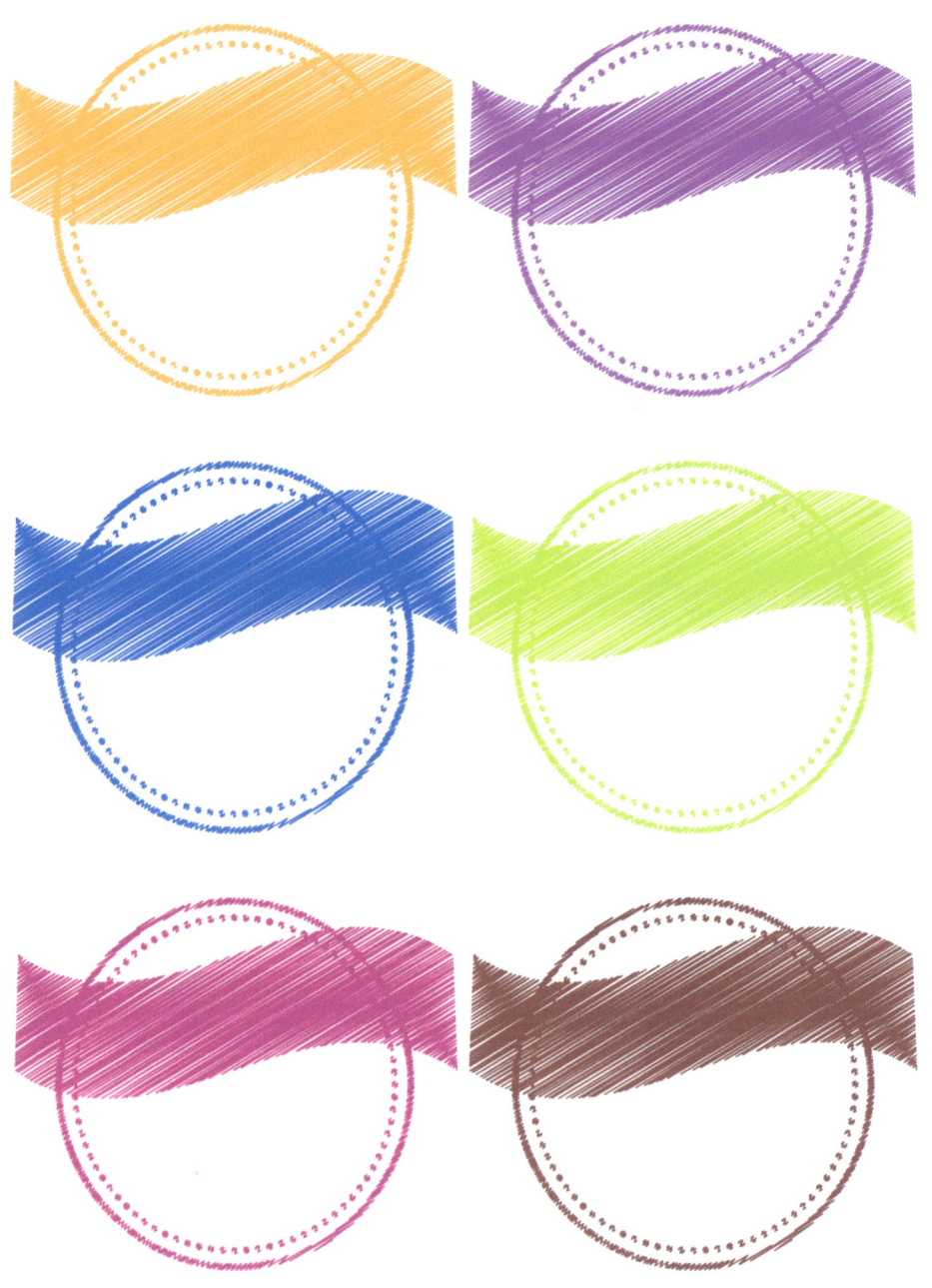

FOOD TRACKER

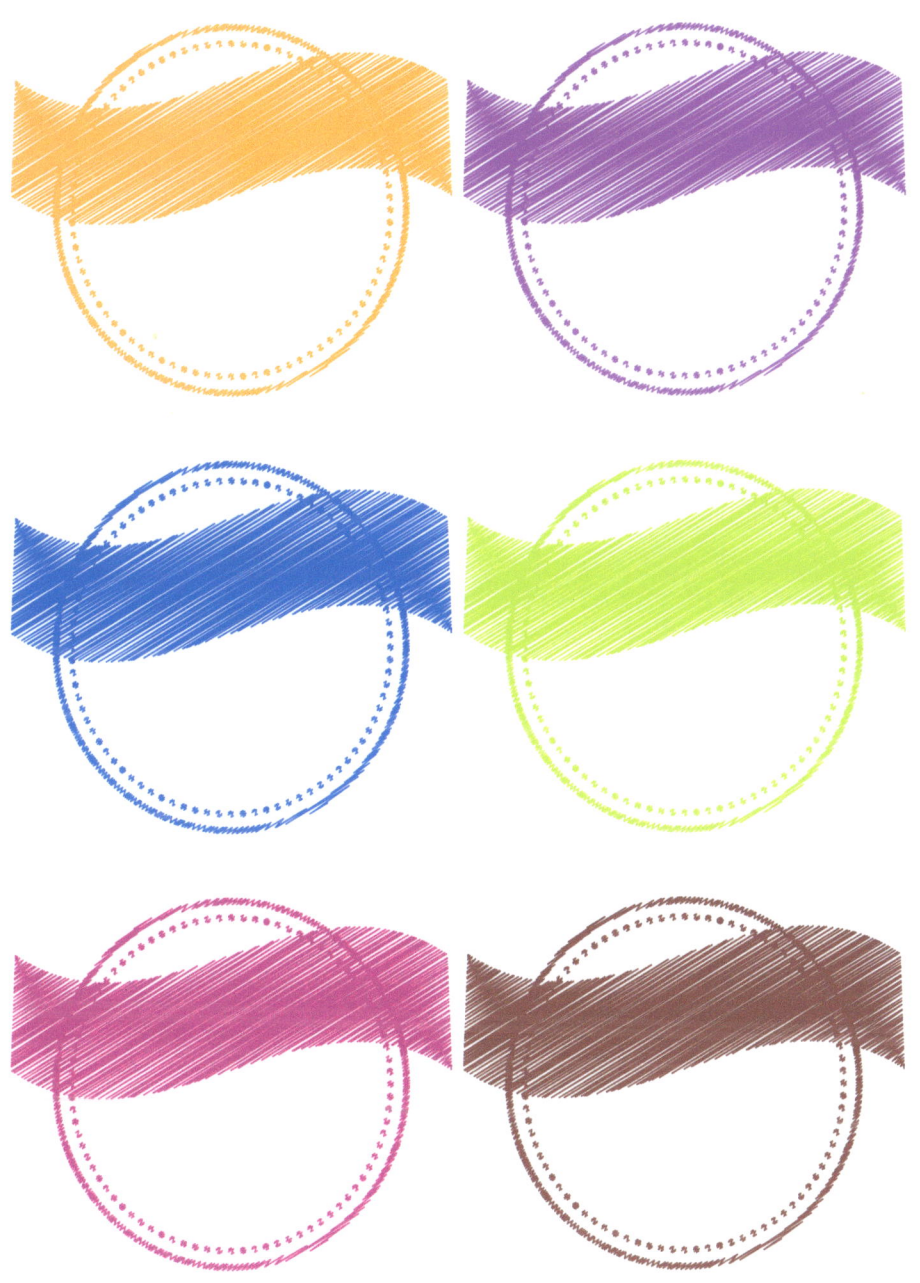

FOOD TRACKER

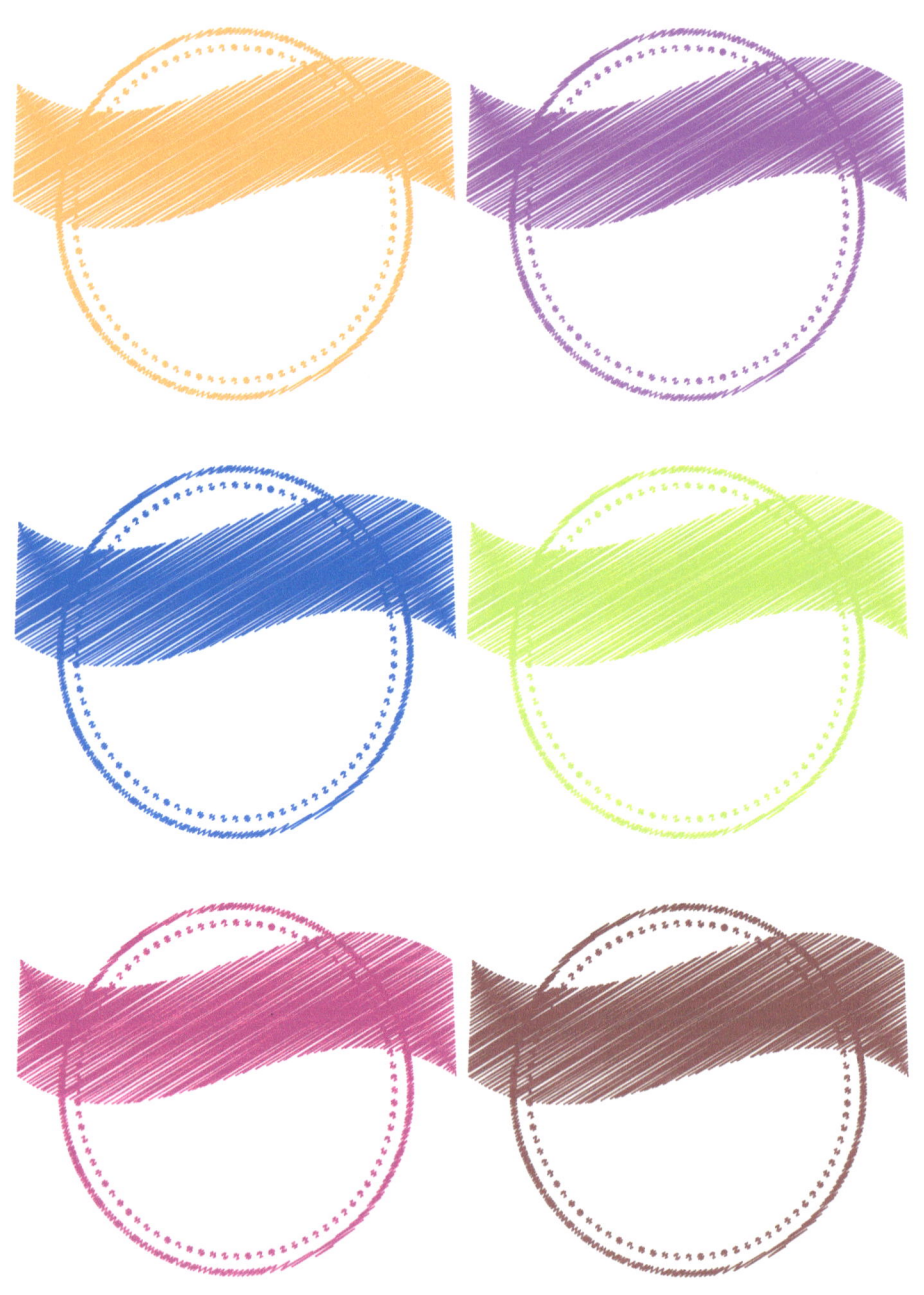

FOOD TRACKER

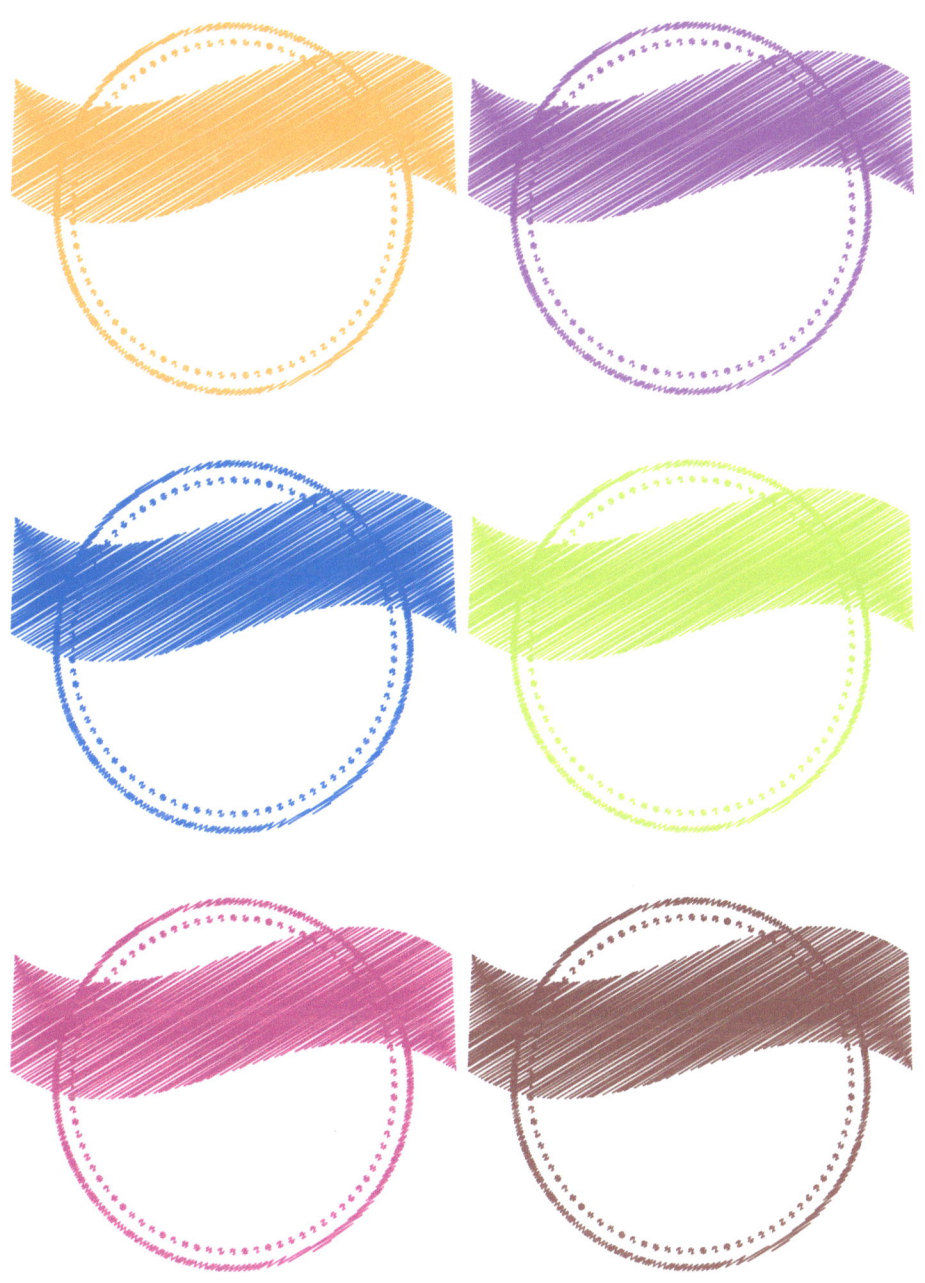

FOOD TRACKER

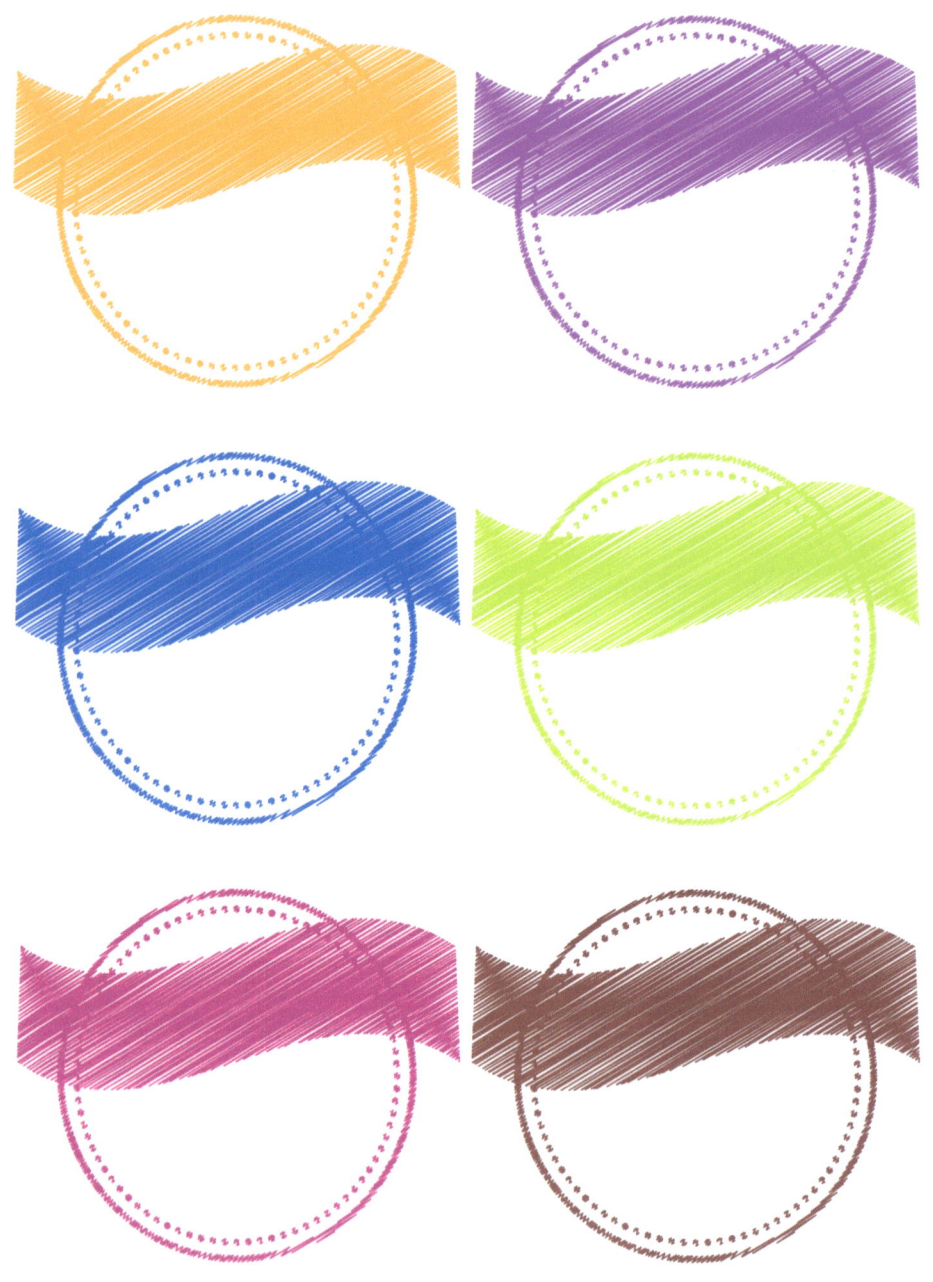

FOOD TRACKER

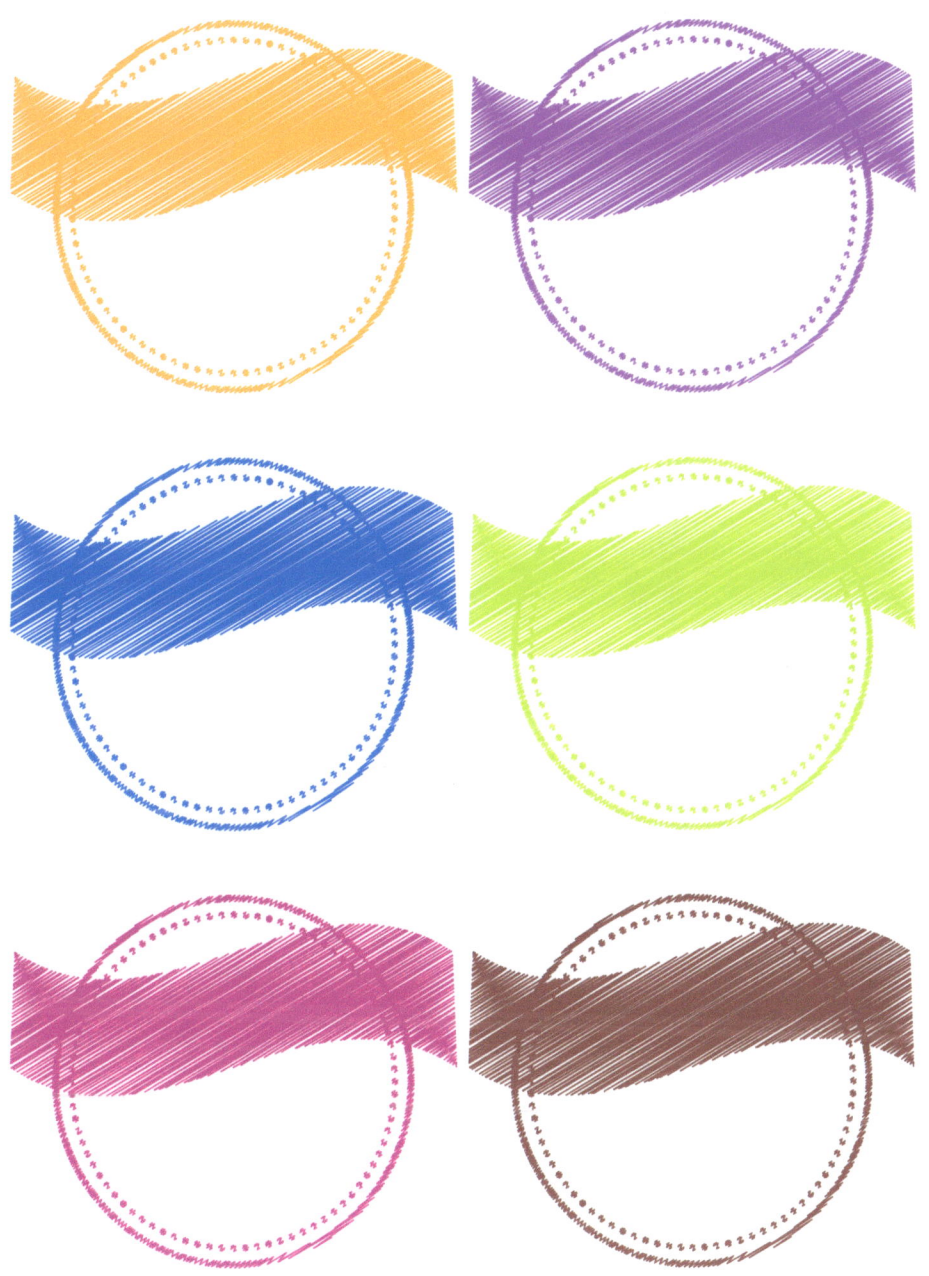

FOOD TRACKER

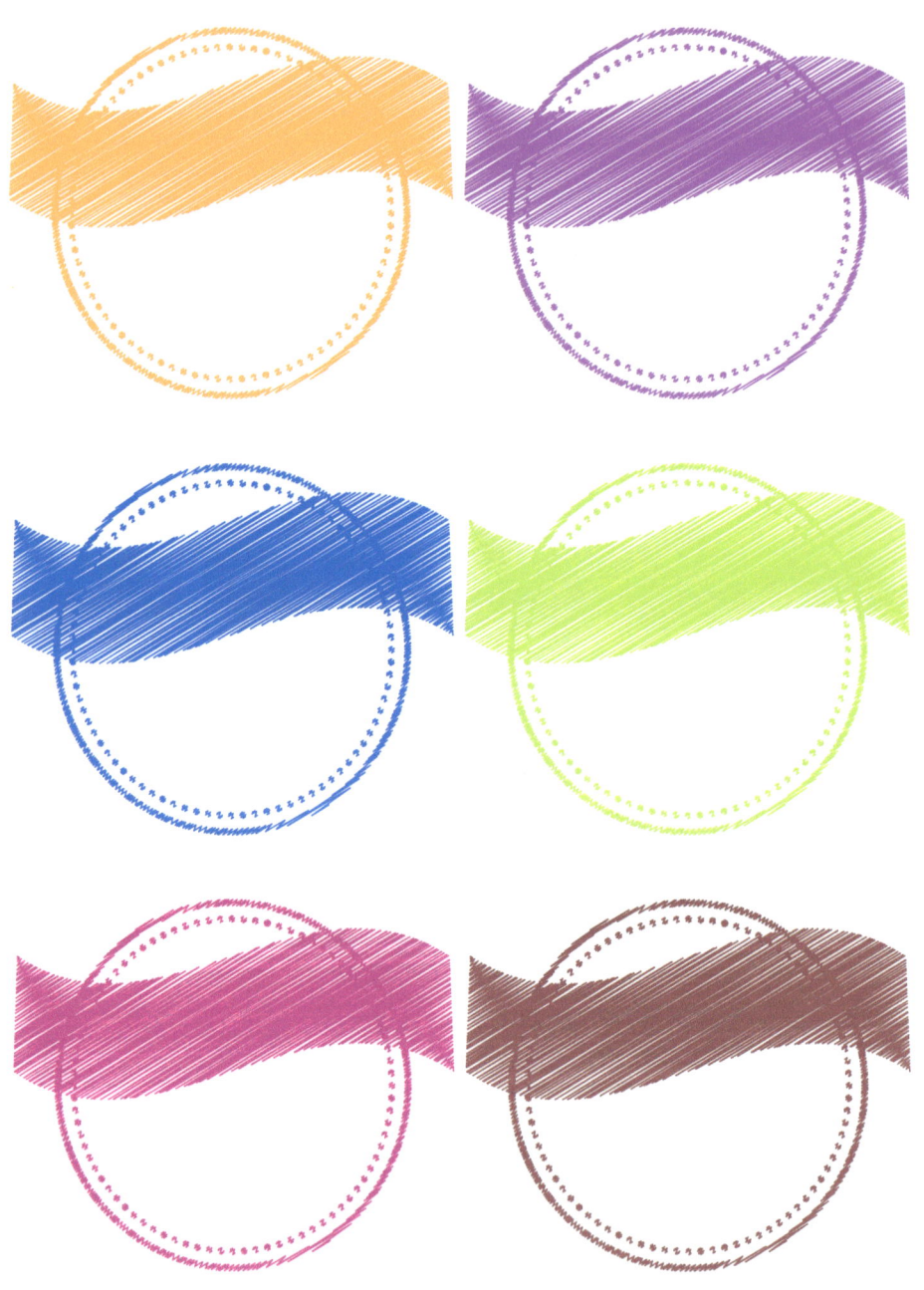

FOOD TRACKER

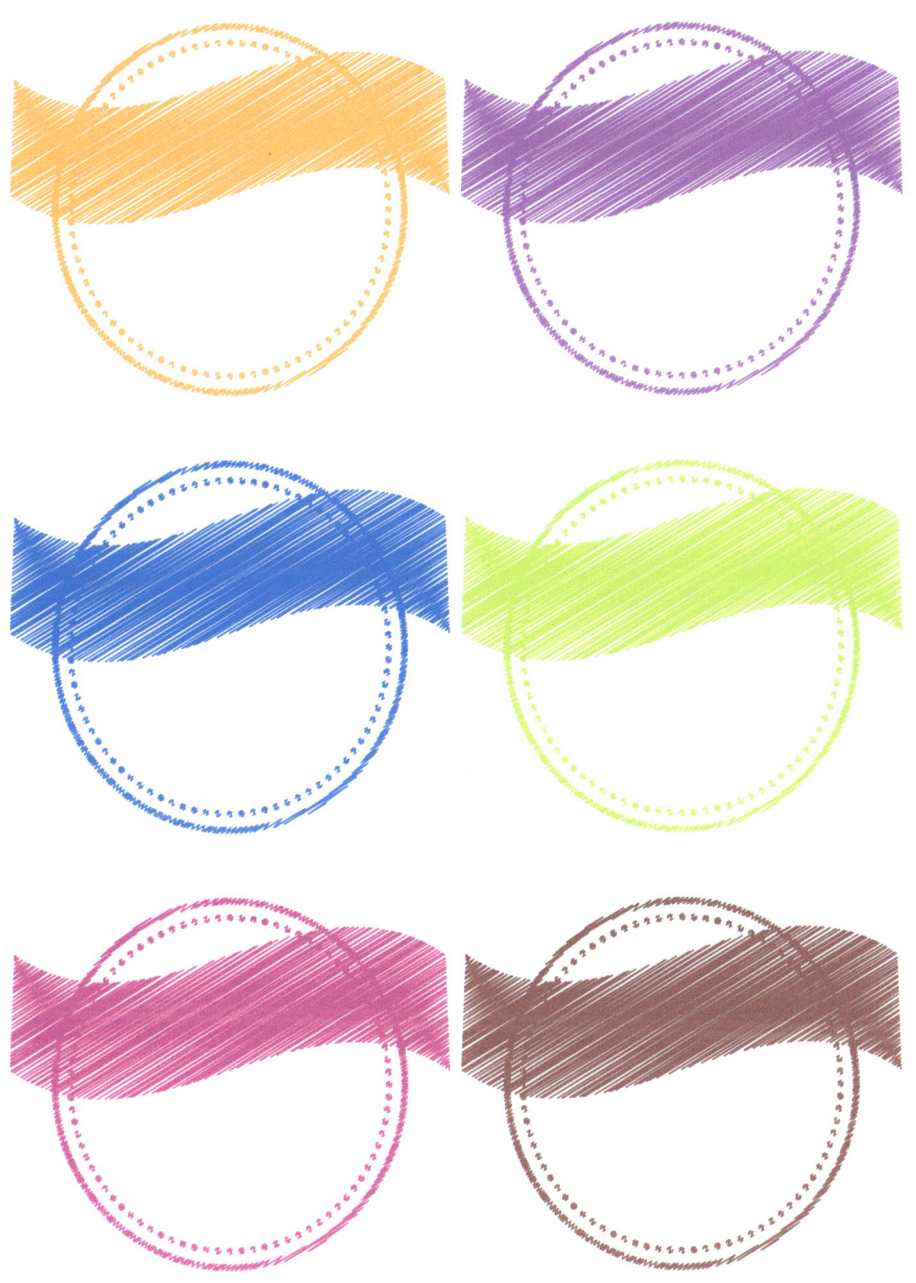

FOOD TRACKER

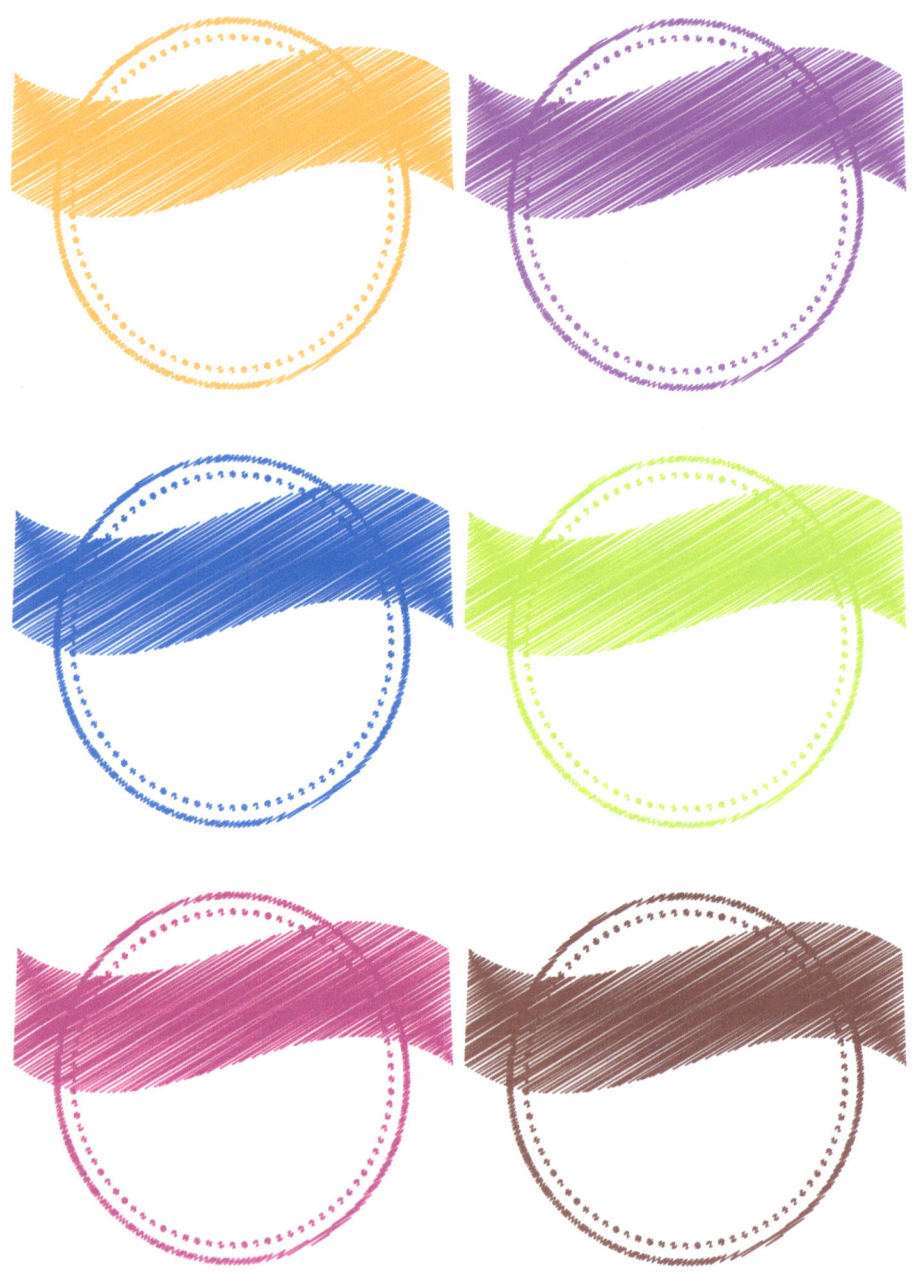

FOOD TRACKER

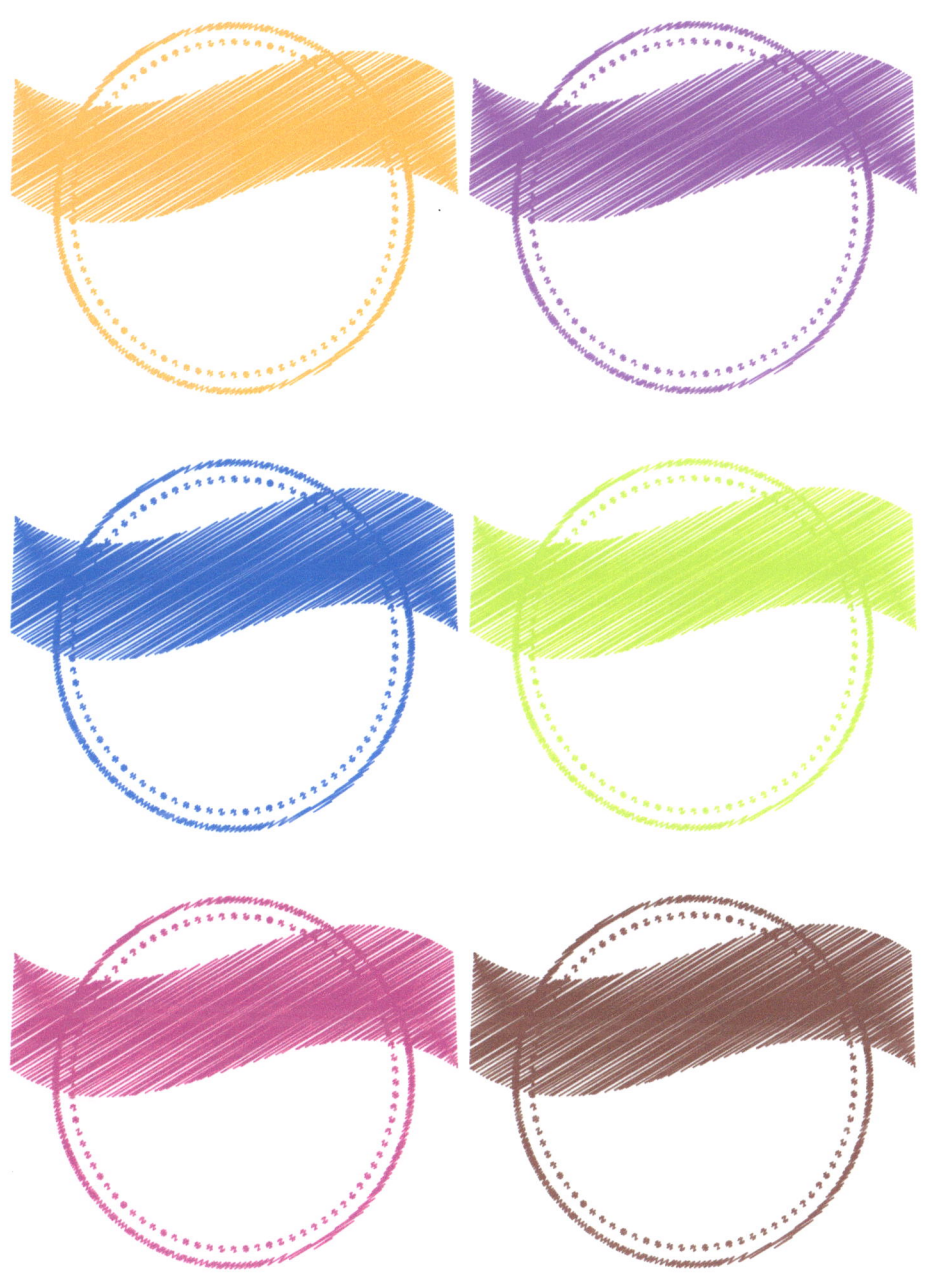

FOOD TRACKER

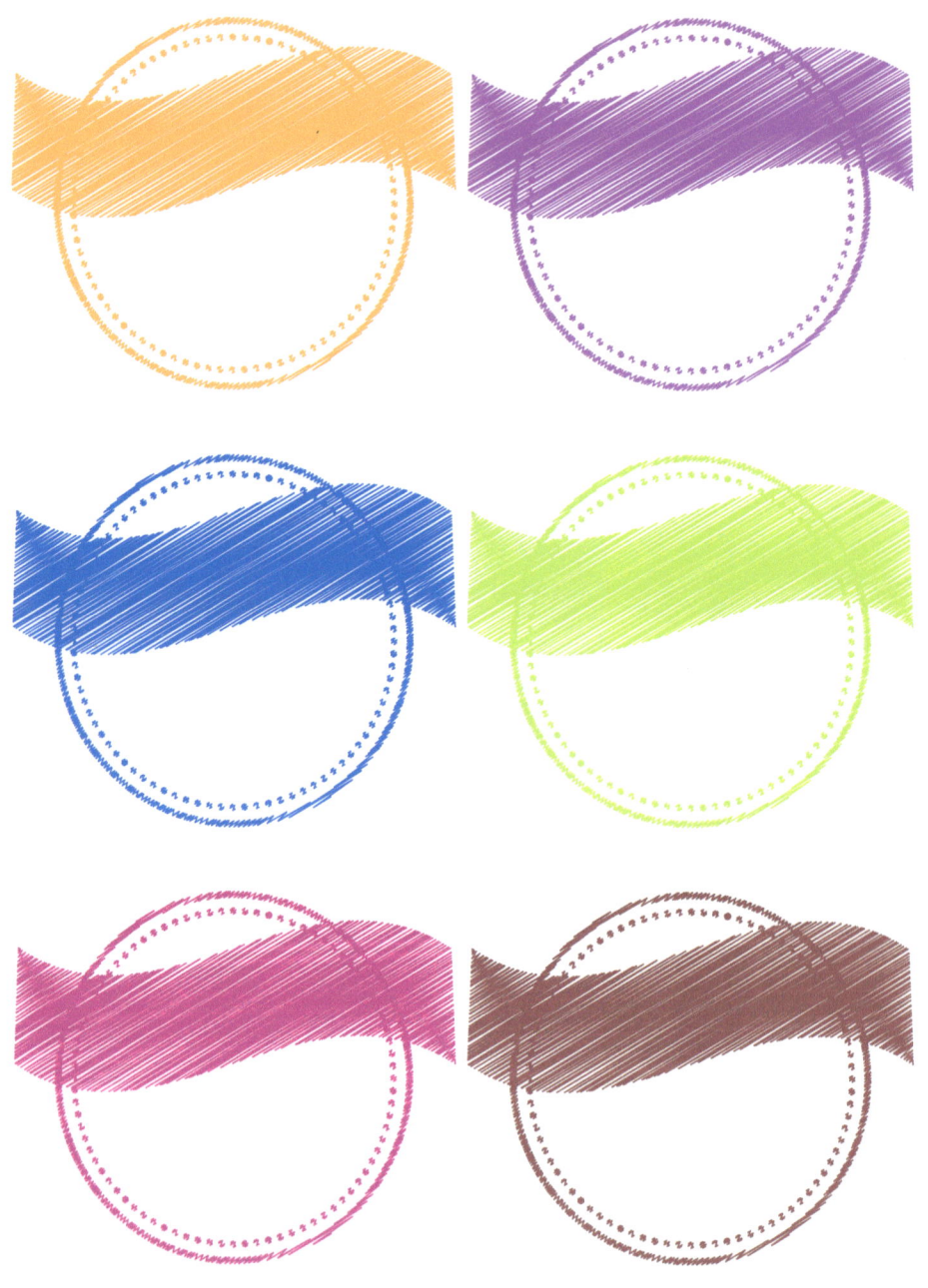